The
S
Diet
Eat Right
Every Time
Guide

DAVID ZINCZENKO

Editor-in-Chief of Men'sHealth.
Author of the *New York Times* bestseller *The Abs Diet*
WITH TED SPIKER

RODALE

This edition first published in the UK in 2005 by
Rodale International Ltd
7–10 Chandos Street
London W1G 9AD
www.rodale.co.uk

© 2005 Rodale Inc.

All rights reserved. No part of this publication may be reproduced or transmitted in any form or by any means, electronic or mechanical, including photocopying, recording or any other information storage and retrieval system, without the written permission of the publisher.

Men's Health is a registered trademark of Rodale Inc.

Printed and bound in the UK by CPI Bath
using acid-free paper from sustainable sources.

1 3 5 7 9 8 6 4 2

Book design by Carol Angstadt

A CIP record for this book is available from the British Library

ISBN 1-4050-8796-X

This paperback edition distributed to the book trade by Pan Macmillan Ltd

Notice
This book is intended as a reference volume only, not as a medical manual. The information given here is designed to help you make informed decisions about your health. It is not intended as a substitute for any treatment that may have been prescribed by your doctor. If you suspect that you have a medical problem, we urge you to seek competent medical help.

Mention of specific companies, organizations or authorities in this book does not imply endorsement by the publisher, nor does mention of specific companies, organizations or authorities imply that they endorse this book.

Whenever possible, I have used published data from major restaurants. Other calculations are based on the standard composition of foods. In cases of similar foods, I examined the nutritional profiles of each and selected one that seemed most representative of an industry-wide standard.

Internet addresses and telephone numbers given in this book were accurate at the time it went to press.

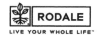

We inspire and enable people to improve their lives and the world around them

Contents

Acknowledgements

SEEING THE ABS DIET come to fruition has been one of the great pleasures of my life. Seeing it make a real impact on the lives of tens of thousands of people has been one of the great rewards. For all of it, I have to thank a number of extraordinarily talented, hard-working and dedicated people who continue to support, encourage and inspire me. In particular:

Steve Murphy, whose courage and commitment to editorial quality has made Rodale Inc. the best publishing company in the world to work for.

The Rodale family, without whom none of this would be possible.

Jeremy Katz, executive editor of *Men's Health* Books, whose wisdom and guidance has made *The Abs Diet* into an extraordinary success.

Ben Roter, whom I want to be when I grow up.

Steve Perrine, who can make a silk purse out of just about anything.

The entire *Men's Health* editorial staff, the smartest and hardest-working group of writers, editors, researchers, designers and photo directors in the industry. Most important, a big shout out to Chris Krogermeier, Marilyn Hauptly, Jennifer Giandomenico, Erin Hobday, Phillip Rhodes, Brenda Miller and everyone else who worked so hard and so fast to publish this book in record time.

My brother, Eric, whose relentless teasing shamed me into taking better care of myself. (Dude, you are sooo dead . . .)

My mother, Janice, who raised two of us nearly single-handedly. Your strength and kindness guide my every action.

My dad, Bohdan, who left this world way too early. I wish you were still here.

Elaine Kaufman, who still lets me order off the menu.

And special thanks also to: Mary Ann Bekkedahl, Michael Bruno, Jeff Csatari, Aimee Geller, Cathy Gruhn, Jon Hammond, Joe Heroun, Samantha Irwin, George Karabotsos, Charlene Lutz, Karen Mazzotta, Patrick McMullan, Peter Moore, Jeff Morgan, Myatt Murphy, Megan Phillips, Scott Quill, Cindy Ratzlaff, Leslie Schneider, Joyce Shirer, Bill Stump, Sara Vigneri, Bug and Fester, and my stepmother, Mickey.

And to Rose. On the rollercoaster of life, you've taught me to let go of the safety bar and reach my hands into the air.

INTRODUCTION

Eat Right Every Time
The Abs Diet Way to a Flat Stomach

DIET IS A FOUR-LETTER word.

That may sound like a strange sentence with which to start a diet book. But then again, this is no ordinary diet book.

We think of a diet as something we 'go on'. A school reunion looms, or a family holiday to the beach is planned, or some other event comes up that tells us it's time to bear down and get rid of that extra layer of flab. And so we do – we 'go on' a diet. Then, once we've lost the desired weight, we 'go off' the diet and back to our old habits of eating cold macaroni cheese while standing over the kitchen sink. Soon enough, another important event looms, and we're back on another diet again. Up and down, up and down goes our weight, but mostly, over time, it goes up. That's because deprivation diets and fads like eating low-fat, eating low-carb or eating nothing but grapefruit just don't work in the long run. In fact, they stress your body so much that your body responds by trying even harder to store fat, especially in the midsection.

A recent study in the *American Journal of Preventive Medicine* found that about 60 per cent of Americans who try to lose weight do so by restricting their calorie intakes, with roughly one in 10 skipping meals in a desperate attempt to strip off the flab. But study after study has shown that yo-yo dieting is one of the best ways to ensure your stomach will get bigger and flabbier in the months and years ahead.

Well, those days are over!

The Abs Diet is a revolutionary new way of eating, one that's helped tens of thousands of people lose hundreds of thousands of kilograms. In fact, with the Abs Diet – a simple, six-times-a-day eating plan that will never let you get hungry – you can lose 4.5 kg/10 lb, 6.8 kg/15 lb, even 9 kg/20 lb, from your tummy first, in 6 weeks or less.

The Abs Diet isn't a traditional diet, because you'll eat so much delicious food – from steak to strawberries, bread to bacon, soup to nuts – that you'll never want or need to stray from it. In fact, if you're ever hungry on the Abs Diet – well, then, you're not on the Abs Diet.

See, I know how hard it is to lose weight using traditional methods. As a boy growing up in small-town Pennsylvania, I too struggled with a weight problem. I made bad choices – choosing fast food over smart food, then trying to starve myself to get my body into the shape I wanted it. Sure enough, I'd get hungry, and there I'd be, barking my lunch order into a clown's mouth once again. My brother, Eric, used to invite his friends over to watch my dietary indiscretions: 'Don't disturb the big animal,' he'd tell his buddies. 'It's feeding.'

But all that's changed. As the editor-in-chief of *Men's Health*, I've spent the past 10 years poring over cutting-edge research in nutrition, fitness, weight loss and exercise. And what I've learned, I've distilled into the Abs Diet – a programme that's been proven time and time again to strip away belly fat and leave you looking and feeling better than ever.

The Secret to Perfect Weight Control Is in Your Hands

THE ABS DIET REVOLVES around a dozen delicious, convenient foods I call the ABS DIET POWER 12. All you need to do is eat the acronym: **A**lmonds and other nuts, **B**eans and other pulses, **S**pinach and other green vegetables, **D**airy (low-fat), **I**nstant (quick-cooking) and other oats, **E**ggs, **T**urkey, other lean meats and fish, **P**eanut butter, **O**live oil, **W**holegrain breads and cereals, **E**xtra-protein (whey) powder, **R**aspberries and other berries.

Yup, you read that right: you get to eat healthy protein, healthy fats, healthy carbs – there's hardly anything you need to give up on this programme. Ice cream? Sure. Grilled cheese sandwiches? Yup. Uncle Frank's famous chilli? You bet. All I want you to do is eat more good food, more often, and maybe make a few small adjustments to the ingredients of your favourites to make them just as delicious – and twice as nutritious. And as for the few foods I do want you to say goodbye to – anything that stains your fingers orange, for example – well, I've come up with some great, tasty, healthy alternatives.

The Abs Diet is so easy even Homer Simpson could handle it. There's no measuring, no counting calories, no complicated equations, no hours-in-the-kitchen recipes. Just simple, smart, delicious food you'll enjoy all day long.

But even though the Abs Diet is simple, modern life is complicated. The supermarkets and chain restaurants are filled with foods that look healthy but really aren't; foods that are packed with high-calorie sweeteners that actually increase your appetite; foods that are greased up with unhealthy, chemically altered fats that clog up your plumbing; and foods that have had all their nutritional value stripped from them before they're wrapped in cellophane and set on the supermarket shelf. And even family life comes fraught with its own perils: in a survey of

274 single and married women by Texas Tech University Health Sciences Center, researchers found that almost 60 per cent of married women were obese, compared to just 43 per cent of singles. 'Women in larger households have four times the odds of being obese in comparison to women who live alone,' says study author James E Rohrer, PhD. He suggests that more people in the household translates into more food in the fridge and a risk of obesity that is four times greater than that of women who live solo.

And that's why I've created this sequel – *The Abs Diet Eat Right Every Time Guide* – to help you make smart, healthy choices on the hoof, whether you're cooking up the family dinner or ordering out on a romantic date. Wherever you may be, *The Abs Diet Eat Right Every Time Guide* will show you how to eat more of the great foods out there and teach you to avoid the fat bombs that are looking to spoil your waistline.

Our relationship with food is a complicated one, especially in the West. Almost half of all British adults are overweight, and 22 per cent are obese (the figures are very similar in Australia, New Zealand and South Africa), and for good reason: we've become people who consider fast food takeaways fine dining, who save money if we order two pizzas instead of one, who love bosses who treat the office to cakes, who've been brainwashed into thinking potatoes are a diet food because they're low in fat, and who build their food pyramids with an order of fried chicken.

With *The Abs Diet Eat Right Every Time Guide*, you'll be armed – literally, to the teeth – with the information you need to make the right choices. I've listed the best foods to buy – and the worst foods to avoid – in hundreds of shopping and eating out situations. Slip this book inside your jacket pocket or into your handbag and be ready whenever, wherever hunger strikes.

Stay Lean – Not Hungry

I TRUST THAT if you've read this far, you're inspired by the idea that you can rebuild your body. But every person who wants to lose fat is motivated by different factors – whether it's because you want to feel better, live longer, look better in a bathing suit, run faster or avoid having your kids mistake you for a Sea World attraction. No matter what your motivation, I think building a diet plan that works into your lifestyle is the most important element for success.

Like I said at the beginning of this book, diet is a four-letter word. It's been twisted around to mean eating less, not eating more or eating better. Say the word and all you see is a 6-month stint of celery sticks and rice cakes. Well, wrong. You should stop thinking about 'dieting' and start thinking about building a healthy 'eating plan'. Even the people you'll read about in this book – people who have lost more than 9 kg/20 lb in 6 weeks – found themselves forgetting about the word *diet*.

Take Jon Armond, who traded in his beer gut for a flat one with a 16-kg/35-lb weight loss in 9 weeks. Jon says he doesn't even miss the foods he used to eat.

'I found myself not even consumed with dieting,' Jon says. 'I've never been on a diet where you didn't have to think about being on the diet all the time.' (See his story on page 82.) That's because the Abs Diet is a system that's easy to follow as it never leaves you hungry and gives you the nutritional balance to have all of your cravings fulfilled.

Eat More – and Weigh Less!

MOST DIETS ARE ABOUT losing – losing meals, losing muscle mass, losing energy. The Abs Diet is about gaining – gaining health and fitness, gaining time and energy, gaining delicious foods you can eat whenever you want. Just look at all you have to gain:

A longer life! Belly fat is the most dangerous kind of fat. That's because it often comprises both subcutaneous fat (fat that's under your skin) and visceral fat (fat that lies beneath your stomach muscles, snug up against your internal organs). It's this second type, visceral fat, that can cause you some long-term harm.

Here's why: in a lean, healthy person, the liver uses both fat and glycogen (i.e., blood sugar) as energy. But if your tummy is hard to the touch and protrudes out in front of you, it means your liver is basically encased in a layer of fat. With so much fat on hand, your liver gets lazy, forgets about glycogen, and just burns fat for energy. Now, normally, burning fat is good – but not without glycogen to balance it. Your liver is like a big iron stove in your living room. You can fill it with clean, dry wood – that's the glycogen. Or you can fill it with rotten fruit, egg shells and polystyrene containers – that's the fat. Both will burn, but one will burn cleanly, and the other will create a horrible, stinky mess.

In your body, that horrible stinky mess is excess cholesterol – the by-product of a liver that burns more fat than glycogen. Perhaps even worse, once your liver gets used to burning fat, it forgets how to properly manage blood sugar. In one report, researchers concluded that visceral fat is the single best predictor of diabetes. So factor in the higher cholesterol, the increased risk of diabetes, and all the complications of the two, and you realize that losing that fat is just as important to your long-term health as losing that eyebrow ring is to your future employment. But that's really only the beginning of the story. Shedding fat from your frame is essential to living long and healthy. Consider:

▶ A Canadian study of 8,000 people found that those with the weakest abdominal muscles (an indicator for fattier abdominal regions) had twice the death rate of those with stronger ones.

▶ Many studies show that men with waists larger than about 88 cm/35 in have an increased risk of heart disease.

▶ A Swedish study found that cancer rates are 33 per cent higher in obese patients than in lean ones.

▶ Overweight men are 50 per cent more likely to develop heart disease, 360 per cent more likely to develop diabetes and 16 per cent more likely to die of a first heart attack.

Bottom line: lose fat, gain years. You don't have to be Albert Einstein to know who gets the better end of that trade.

More and better sex! Sure, losing weight can turn you from a clown to a Clooney, from a jelly baby to an Angelina Jolie. But besides the side effects of looking and feeling better (which gives you more confidence and makes you more attractive to others), losing fat helps with the mechanics of sex. Being overweight makes you 50 per cent more likely to have erectile dysfunction. Of course, there are many factors that control sexual dysfunction in both men and women, but one of the major ones is a supply-and-demand issue. See, when you're sexually excited, your brain sends an all-points bulletin to your pants. *Wet bathing suit ahead, prepare for engagement.* With that message, your brain sends blood downwards to cause an erection in a man or stimulate arousal-sensing and lubricating organs in a woman. But when you're overweight, the after-effects of the afternoon's burger gum up your blood vessels and thus narrow the arteries that lead to Shangri La. Without a sufficient blood supply, nothing happens. If there's no fuel in the tank, your car ain't going anywhere.

A pain-free and injury-proof life! While the core goal of this book is to help you decipher the tricky menu mines you'll encounter through life, another important part of the Abs Diet is transforming your body with a modest amount of exercise. That will teach your body to grow and maintain lean muscle mass. I'll review the workout principles briefly in Chapter 11, but as part of the plan, you'll be doing some work to strengthen your abdominal region. That is, you'll teach your abdominal muscles to be strong. That's not just so you can win a modelling contract. That's because strong abdominal muscles are the infrastructure of your body. Your abs play a role in just about every physical movement you make. They help you run, lift, have sex, stretch, bend, pick up your kids and shimmy through clothes racks. But most importantly, they act – along with your lower back – as your internal girdle to support you through the everyday rigours of life. One US Army study showed that those people with the strongest abdominal muscles were the least likely to be injured (for all kinds of injuries, not just lower-back ones), and that points to the crucial role that strong abdominal muscles play. Strong abdominal muscles will help prevent and alleviate back pain – one of the most debilitating and most common injuries for both men and women.

It helps to realize that abdominal muscles don't really work in isolation; they work as a cohesive group that crisscrosses your midsection and attaches to your spine. When abdominal muscles are weak, other muscles in your body have to pick up the slack. They end up overcompensating, and they end up causing back pain and strain or even more serious back problems.

Abs! If you haven't figured it by now, Sherlock, then let me explain: this programme is about living a healthier life. It'll help you lose weight, it'll help you gain control of what you eat, and it'll help turn your body into a fat-burning, muscle-building juggernaut. Ultimately, this book is about striving to meet your individual goals and looking the way you want to look, and that's where the abs come in. Abs are the by-product of your new outlook on eating and exercising. They're the reward for following a plan that makes you healthier. Of course, if you're one bonbon away from a total couch collapse, it's going to take you a little longer than someone who's only 6 or 7 kg/about 1 stone over their ideal weight. (The typical standard for men is that you need to have a body-fat percentage of around 10 per cent to have visible abs. For women, it's around 14 per cent.) The fact is, everyone has abs, and everyone has the potential to see their abs. It's just a matter of banishing the fat off your gut so you can. Certainly, some people are blessed with high-quality genetics, metabolism or lipo docs, but the potential is there for everyone.

Turn Fat into Muscle!

MOST DIET PLANS DEPEND on willpower for success. The Abs Diet, on the other hand, recruits an often untapped but highly potent ally in your search for slim – your own body!

See, one of the most potent fat-burners around is lurking right below your own skin. It's muscle, and building more can turn your body into a fat-burning machine. For each 455 g/1 lb of muscle you build, you'll burn an extra 50 calories a day – just sitting still. If you were to build just 4.5 kg/10 lb of new muscle, you'd burn off enough extra calories to drop 22.6 kg/50 lb of fat in 1 year – again, simply by sitting still.

Of course, you can't build that muscle by sitting still. So I've included in this book a super-simple workout built around an easy weight-training programme that anyone can do. It won't turn you into a gym rat, the Incredible Hulk or Arnie Schwarzenegger. But it will help you trade flab for lean, sexy muscle. (Feeling eager? Turn to page 179 for a quick peek at the Abs Diet Workout.)

Take Back Control of Your Body – And Your Life!

YOU DON'T HAVE TO just take my word for it. Listen to other people who've embraced the Abs Diet – people like Linda Toomey, who lost 9 kg/20 lb in 6 weeks, while caring for four small children; or Jim Phillips, who was stuck in a weight rut for years until he found this revolutionary and easy plan; or Kyle Snay, who lost more than 9 kg/20 lb on the programme and alleviated all of his back pain while doing so. As of now, there are more than 100,000 people taking the Abs Diet Challenge (you can find it on www.absdiet.com). The stories of the many people who have tried and succeeded on the Abs Diet show the power of the plan.

Now, with *The Abs Diet Eat Right Every Time Guide*, you have a passport to success no matter where you and your stomach may wander. What I want is for you to use the Abs Diet Powerfoods as the guiding philosophy for the way you eat. With more than 100 recipes in this book, you'll cook up plenty of tasty ways to help you lose fat. But I also want you to use this guide to help you manage situations when you face more tough questions than Michael Jackson's publicist. It's one thing to eat right when you prepare the foods yourself; it's quite another when you're at the mercy of lard-slinging chefs.

Above all – and this is really the foundation for *Eat Right Every Time* – I want you to feel one way while taking part in the Abs Diet: satisfied.

Satisfied . . . that you'll never be hungry.

Satisfied . . . that you won't be denied great-tasting foods.

Satisfied . . . that you have the flexibility to eat according to your lifestyle.

Satisfied . . . that you'll have the knowledge to eat right anywhere you go.

Satisfied . . . that the only new trousers you'll ever have to buy will be smaller.

Satisfied – make that ecstatic – with your new body!

THE ABS DIET
CHEAT SHEET

THIS AT-A-GLANCE GUIDE summarizes the principles of the Abs Diet: the 6-week plan to flatten your stomach and keep you lean for life.

SUBJECT	GUIDELINE
Number of meals	Six a day, spaced relatively evenly throughout the day. Eat snacks 2 hours before larger meals.
The **ABS DIET POWER 12**	Base most meals on these groups of foods. Every meal should have at least two foods from the list.
	Almonds and other nuts **B**eans and pulses **S**pinach and other green vegetables
	Dairy (fat-free or low-fat milk, yogurt, cheese) **I**nstant oats (unsweetened, unflavoured) **E**ggs **T**urkey, other lean meats and fish
	Peanut butter **O**live oil **W**holegrain breads and cereals **E**xtra-protein (whey) powder **R**aspberries and other berries
Portion size	While many diets are based on controlling portion size, the Abs Diet is designed to be self-controlling. The high-fibre, high-protein foods you'll encounter in this book will fill you up and keep you feeling full for hours. Your body will tell you when it's time to eat – and when it's time to stop.

SUBJECT	GUIDELINE
Secret weapons	Each of the ABS DIET POWER 12 has been chosen in part for its stealthy, healthy secret weapons – the nutrients that will help power up your natural fat burners, protect you from illness and injury, and keep you lean and fit for life!
Nutritional ingredients to emphasize	Protein, monounsaturated and polyunsaturated fats, fibre, calcium.
Nutritional ingredients to limit	Refined carbohydrates (or carbs with high glycaemic index), saturated fats, trans fats, glucose syrup.
Alcohol	Limit yourself to two or three drinks per week, to maximize the benefits of the Abs Diet plan.
Ultimate Powerfood	Smoothies. The combination of the calcium and protein in milk, yogurt and whey powder, combined with the fibre in oats and fruit, makes them one of the more filling and easy options.
Cheating	One meal a week, eat anything you want.
Exercise programme	Optional for the first 2 weeks. Weeks 3 to 6 incorporate a 20-minute, full-body workout 3 days a week. Emphasis is on strength training, brisk walking and some abdominal work.
At-home workout	Gym workouts and at-home workouts are both detailed to excuse-proof your fitness plan.
Abdominal workout	At the beginning of two of your strength-training workouts. One exercise for each of the five different parts of your abs.

ABS DIET SUCCESS STORY

INSPIRED TO LOSE, INSPIRED TO WIN

Name: Bret Freeman

Age: 38

Height: 1.77 m/5'10"

Weight, Week 1: 93 kg/14 st 9 lb

Weight, Week 6: 83 kg/13 st 1 lb

Weight, Week 17: 79.5 kg/12 st 7 lb

'I was just basically tired of being a fat slob,' says Bret Freeman, who had been a lean, fit wrestler at school but had steadily gained weight over the years.

'I tried Atkins and all the fad diets out there. I'd go on and off, and it always seemed like I gained back more weight than what I started out with,' says Freeman, who once reached an all-time high of 111 kg/17 st 7 lb. 'I tried The Zone diet, and that thing was so dang complicated; you had to put so much thought into what you ate, good sugars and bad sugars, what it did to your insulin levels. It was horrible.'

When Freeman heard about how simple the Abs Diet was, he couldn't wait to get started. So he read it through in a day and a half and started the following Monday. At the same time, he bought a home gym and started the exercise programme. The weight started coming off immediately.

'I think the Abs Diet worked for me for a combination of reasons, but one was that it kept me eating delicious food all day long,' he says. 'People would notice how much weight I lost, and they'd say, "You must be starving yourself." And I'd tell them, "You wouldn't believe how much I eat." '

The change? Besides the weight, Freeman lost inches. He started the diet in snug 38s, and now his 32s are a little loose. 'I think I'm ready to go down to a 30.' Motivated by Lance Armstrong's story, he's now set to do a couple of triathlons, and he's been asked to be the head coach for the school wrestling team. Plus, there's the added satisfaction he feels when he goes to his sons' football games, where he hasn't seen other parents since last season. Freeman says, 'One friend joked that they saw my wife, and they thought she had a new husband because I looked so different.'

And in a way, she did.

Chapter I

YOUR WEIGHT IS REALLY NOT YOUR FAULT

EVERYONE HAS ENEMIES. Batman has the Joker. Spiderman has the Green Goblin. Joan Rivers has gravity. You? Sure, your neighbour may slice your perennials when he mows the lawn, and the boss's henchman may boil your blood, but to me, the biggest enemies you face are the profiteering junk-food merchants of the food industry.

In a time-strapped society and in your time-strapped life, these piranhas prey on consumers who need a quick fix – a quick fix of fat, fries and foods designed to hypnotize you with their taste and stretch you at your waist. As you surely can see at any shopping centre food court or stretch of commercialized suburbia, we live in a world of fast food. We have a world rich with hot dog vendors, pizza windows, order-at-the-counter restaurants, chain restaurants and extra-value meals – a world where, even when you want to eat healthily, it sometimes feels impossible to do so.

These places pelt you with chips, suffocate your innards with ice cream and shoot chocolate-coated peanuts into your mouth.

But fast food doesn't need to be fat food. Convenient eating doesn't have to mean that fat conveniently claims squatter's rights on your gut. Easy eating doesn't mean greasy eating.

The secret of the Abs Diet's success is that you can follow it no matter where you are. If you just remember to eat the acronym – the ABS DIET POWER 12 – you'll stay lean, fit and healthy no matter where you are. You don't have to fall victim to kitchens that have more grease than a mechanic's fingernails, and you don't have to stop enjoying the taste of food to do so.

You can eat fast.

You can enjoy what you eat.

And you can be free from hunger, deprivation and culinary boredom.

I want to arm you with the information you need to make smart decisions about eating on the go or on a Friday family night out. Before I explain the Abs Diet plan and give you hundreds of choices for what to eat no matter what situation you're in, it's important to review your nutritional friends and enemies. There are only a few things that you can do to fundamentally change the way your body's chemicals, hormones and organs function, but the one major thing that you do that changes your body's internal systems is eat. Ultimately, your health is dictated by the nutrients that travel through your bloodstream after you've put them in your mouth. Here's a quick primer on the pitfalls of your nutritional world.

Your Enemies

The Hunger-Booster: High-Fructose Corn Syrup (HFCS)

I believe there's one primary reason why many people fail on diets – and why they eat poorly to begin with. They're so damn hungry.

Sound simple? Anatomically, it's a little more complicated. And the complication has come in the form of a little-known but shockingly ubiquitous food additive called High-Fructose Corn Syrup (HFCS).

Never heard of HFCS? Then you'll be even more shocked by this next fact: the average American consumes almost 29 kg/63 lb of it each year, and consumers elsewhere don't lag far behind.

Sit and think about that for a moment. Sixty-two pounds of it each year – or about 228 extra calories every day – and you don't even know what it is.

And you're not going to be any happier once you find out: see, up until the 1970s, most sweets were made with simple white sugar. Bad for you, but it was what it was. You sated your sweet tooth, your body absorbed the calories, and you got full pretty fast. But about three decades ago, food manufacturers discovered an easier way to make fizzy drinks, cereals, yogurts and some 40,000 more manufactured foods taste sweeter. They developed HFCS, which is derived from corn and is many times cheaper – and sweeter – than simple sugar. Today, HFCS is added to a shocking number of foods, including foods you wouldn't equate with sweeteners: ketchup, pasta sauce, even crackers. And it's screwing up our metabolic system.

Mechanically, the system works like this: when you eat any type of carbohydrate (like bread or fruit), your body releases insulin to regulate your body weight – pushing those carb calories into your muscles to be used as energy or storing them for later use. Then, like a shut-off mechanism on a petrol pump, it suppresses your appetite. That's the signal that tells your body to stop filling; your tank is full.

The problem is that fructose doesn't stimulate insulin anywhere like as much as regular sugar (sucrose) does, so your body doesn't register it the way it registers simple white sugar. That's why it's possible to see people drink 2-litre bottles of soft drinks in a single sitting. Thirty years ago, that would have been an impossible task, but today, HFCS makes the same number of calories go down and, incredibly, still leaves you hungry for more. Your muscles still need energy, so you crave more food and more sweets. And so you eat more foods containing HFCS, and the cycle continues. Less energy, more flab. HFCS could well stand for Here's Flab Coming to your Stomach.

You don't need to eliminate this artificial foodstuff from your diet entirely, but you need to ensure your meals don't revolve around it, as many people's do. So start checking the food labels: if HFCS is listed first or second on the ingredients list, look at the chart on the nutrition label to see how much sugar the food contains. If it's just a gram or two, it's fine. But if you see a food that has 8 or more grams of sugar, and HFCS is prominent on the list of ingredients, it's a sign that you should leave it on the shelf.

FOODS HIGH IN HFCS OR FRUCTOSE	REPLACE WITH
Regular soft drinks	Unsweetened sparkling water or diet drinks
Commercial sweets (such as jelly beans)	Chocolate (check the label; some chocolate bars have HFCS)
Pancake syrup	Pure maple syrup
Frozen yogurt	Ice cream
Fruit-flavoured yogurt	Artificially sweetened, sugar-sweetened or, best of all, organic yogurt
Highly sweetened cereals	Sugar-free or low-sugar cereals
Pasta sauce	Sugar-free pasta sauce

The Artery Hardener: Trans Fat

If High-Fructose Corn Syrup is Bonnie, then trans fat is Clyde, because together, the duo is responsible for some seriously heinous crimes against your body.

Firstly, it's important to know that dietary fats are a little like college bands, minus the long hair and low trousers. Some are actually good, and some are unbelievably bad. Trans fat falls into the latter category. Trans fat increases the amount of bad cholesterol in your body, for example, and has been linked to an increased risk of heart disease, diabetes and a weakened immune system. Scientists have estimated that trans fat contributes to more than 30,000 premature deaths every year.

So what exactly is this stuff? Once again, it's a Frankenstein monster that's come lumbering out of the labs of the food industry.

Trans fat is created by combining vegetable oil (a liquid) with hydrogen to create partially hydrogenated oil, or trans fatty acids. Once infused with hydrogen, liquid vegetable oil turns into a solid at room temperature, becoming what we recognize today as margarine and yellow spreads.

Trans fats are beloved by the food and restaurant industries for several reasons. Number one, they're cheap. Number two, they can stick around seemingly forever without going bad. (How gross is that?) Number three, you can add them to myriad foods in a way you can't add regular oil – a cookie with vegetable oil in it will ooze all over the supermarket shelf, but one with partially hydrogenated oil in it will stay crisp and tantalizing. So it's no surprise that food marketers, eager to deliver the sensuous flavour and mouth feel of fat to millions of unsuspecting consumers, now add partially hydrogenated oils to all sorts of things – crisps (potato chips), frozen foods, cakes, confectionery, to name a few.

But think about what trans fats are: fats that are supposed to be liquid but are turned into solids. Now think about what they do when they get inside you. Instead of melting like they would in their natural state, they try to revert to their waxy, solid nature. Once you understand that heart disease and stroke are caused in part by waxy build-ups of fat solids in the circulatory system, it's easy to put two and two together. Turning oils into solids isn't doing us a favour – not by a long run.

In America, the US government is finally recognizing the dangers of trans fats. In 2003, food companies were required to list these trans fats for the first time. In the UK, however, the government has, as yet, no plans to implement this, though as consumers become more interested in what is in their food such a change is possible. In the meantime, use these tactics to reduce your intake of trans fats:

▶ Check the ingredient list for 'hydrogenated' or 'partially hydrogenated'. The higher these ingredients are on the label, the more trans fats they contain.

▶ Decode the food label. For those products that don't list trans fats, add all the fat grams together that are listed on the label and then subtract that number from the total fat content. The number you're left with is the estimate for the amount of trans fat.

▶ Snack on baked crisps (potato chips) instead of ones fried in vegetable oil (check the ingredients list).

▶ Pick high-protein breakfasts like eggs or lean bacon instead of waffles. If you have toast, use jam instead of margarine.

▶ At a restaurant, ask what kind of oil the chef uses. You want to hear olive oil.

▶ When eating dinner out, avoid bread, which may be made with trans fats. It's better to pick a baked potato, soup or a salad.

▶ Blot oil from your chips as quickly as possible. A napkin can absorb excess grease.

IF YOU WANT	PICK THIS TRANS FAT-FREE OPTION
Biscuits	Pure butter shortbread (some gingernuts, oat cakes and digestive biscuits are OK too – check the label)
Chocolate	Green & Black's chocolate
Crackers	Ryvita Multigrain crackers

French fries	McCain Oven Chips
Potato chips/crisps	Ruffles Natural sea-salted, reduced-fat crisps

The Belly Buster: Saturated Fats

Just the name sounds threatening, doesn't it? Saturated fats, as in they're going to sink into your stomach and saturate your organs with soft little globs of putty. Bleeech!

And the truth is just as gross as you imagine it to be. Your body likes to burn some kinds of fats – polyunsaturated (from vegetables) and monounsaturated (from nuts and seeds) fats – as energy. But your body would rather save saturated fats around your tummy to use for future energy in case, I dunno, your plane crashes in the jungles of the Philippines or something. Assuming there's no Bataan Death March in your immediate future, however, your body will continue to hold onto the fat it's stored, and the more you eat, the more you wear. Besides raising cholesterol rates, saturated fats have also been shown to increase your risk of heart disease and some types of cancer.

Saturated fats are found primarily in meats and dairy products. 'But wait!' you say. 'Aren't meats and dairy products part of the ABS DIET POWER 12?' Yes, and that's why I emphasize lean meats like turkey, chicken and some cuts of beef, and recommend that you look for low-fat dairy products like low-fat milk or low-fat yogurt whenever possible. The trick is to get the most nutrients – muscle-building protein and fat-fighting calcium – with the least amount of saturated fats.

The Energy Sucker: Refined Carbohydrates

Consider the simple wheat stalk: there it stands, soaking up the sun and minding its own business, a single droplet in a vast sea of amber waves. Who'd have thought this humble grain would spark a controversy more complicated than the JFK assassination? And yet the dietary landscape is wrought by forces arguing grains' place at our dinner table. On one side, the traditional food guide pyramid, which calls for six to eleven servings of grains a day. And on the other side, the Atkins addicts and other no-carb adherents

HOW METABOLISM WORKS – AND HOW TO MAKE IT WORK FOR YOU

Even if you're lying in bed, lounging on the sofa, or sitting on the toilet as you're reading this, your body is burning calories. It's burning calories to keep your heart beating, your lungs breathing, your brain dreaming about lying on a beach in Barbados . . . Hey, wake up!

That calorie burn I'm referring to is your metabolism, and how high it's revving is what determines whether you're losing fat right now – or gaining it. See, your body burns calories all the time, and it burns them in three different ways. One, you burn them when you eat, simply through the act of digestion (remember, it takes more energy to digest protein than it does carbs). Two, you burn calories by exercise and movement, whether you're running a marathon or just walking down the hall. And the last way you burn calories is when you're at rest; that's called your *basal metabolism*, and it refers to the way your body uses fuel when you're not doing anything. Incredibly enough, this is when the majority of your calories are burned – while you're doing nothing.

That explains, in part, why watching those calories tick away on the treadmill or the exercise bike is an exercise in frustration. If the majority of calories are burned during your non-exercising times, then it makes sense to boost your calorie burn during those times, and the way you do that is by adding muscle. In fact, for every 455 g/1 lb of muscle you build, your body will need to burn off up to 50 extra calories a day, just sitting around doing nothing. Add 2.75 kg/6 lb of muscle, and you're burning up to 300 extra calories a day, just hanging out being you.

Later on in this book, I'll walk you through the basics of the Abs Diet Workout, a muscle-building, fat-burning, 20-minute workout that will help you create the body you've always wanted.

who believe that simple stalk of wheat is evil incarnate.

The truth is . . . well, the truth is in neither corner, but some-where more towards the middle.

The truth is that the human body can't survive without car-bohydrates, because grains – like fruits, vegetables and other carbs – provide crucial energy to feed the brain, the muscles and the metabolism. Grains also provide crucial vitamins, minerals and fibre, all of which the body needs to stay healthy. For exam-ple, a recent study at Brigham and Women's Hospital in Boston found that women who consumed 800 or more micrograms of folic acid a day had 29 per cent less risk of high blood pressure than those who consumed less than 200 micrograms daily. Folic acid is just one of the many nutrients found in carbohydrates.

But the anti-carb movement does have its points to make, because most of the carbohydrates in our diet aren't rich in all those great nutrients and fibre. They're 'refined carbohydrates', such as white sugar, white bread, bagels, biscuits, et cetera. Most baked goods, in fact, are made from grains that have had all their great nutrients 'refined' out of them.

This causes serious problems for the carb lover. A slice of bread made with whole grains – wheat, oats, or what have you – is full of fibre. Fibre expands once it's in the stomach, taking up space, slow-ing the digestive process, and keeping your energy and hunger lev-els even for several hours. Take out the fibre, though, and those carb calories go shooting through the digestive tract faster than Bill Clinton at a sorority party. There's a rush of blood sugar as the carbs are quickly digested, a burst of energy, and then a letdown as insulin stores the blood sugar and your body cries out for more.

That's why the ABS DIET POWER 12 includes wholegrain breads and cereals, along with fruit, vegetables and other carbohy-drate sources. Carbs have the energy you need; you just have to choose wisely. Read the label; you want to see the words 'whole grain' on your bread, cereal and cracker boxes whenever possible.

Your Friends

The Muscle Builder: Protein

You may think of protein as the staple ingredient for bodybuilders or the Atkins crowd, but protein has more super powers than the High Court. For one, protein helps kick-start your metabolism. It takes your body twice as much energy to break down protein as it does to break down carbohydrates, so when you eat a high-protein meal, you actually burn off additional calories at the dinner table. In one study, for example, people who ate a high-protein diet burned more than twice as many calories in the hours after their meals as people on a high-carbohydrate diet.

Protein also flips your satisfaction switch. When you start your meal with protein – say, downing a glass of skimmed milk before breakfast or ordering the prawn cocktail appetizer at dinner – your body registers its satiation level earlier on, and you wind up eating less. And that effect can carry on throughout the day. Some studies have shown that, if all calories are equal, people who eat a high-protein meal feel fuller and eat less at their next meal than those who don't. In another study, subjects who followed a high-protein diet lost an average of 9 kg/20 lb each, compared to just 5 kg/11 lb lost by participants who followed a low-protein diet. Amazingly, protein not only burned away fat, it burned away tummy fat. The high-protein dieters lost twice as much abdominal fat as their low-protein dieting counterparts.

The Cholesterol Cutters: Polyunsaturated and Monounsaturated Fats

Ten years ago, if I had told you to eat more fat, I'd have been dragged from my office by the diet police and run out of town. Although it's generally a good idea to cut down on some kinds of fats – like trans fats and saturated fats – other kinds are actually good for you. Good? Heck, they're great.

Our bodies need fat. We need it to deliver vitamins throughout our bodies. We need it to produce testosterone – the hormone that leads to muscle growth. And we need it to keep satiated and full. In fact, one of the important things we've learned recently is that reducing your fat intake doesn't necessarily decrease your body-fat percentage over the long haul. In a recent study at Brigham and Women's Hospital in Boston, participants were put on either a low-fat or moderate-fat diet. After 6 months, the two groups lost about the same amount of weight. But when doctors checked in

ABS DIET SUCCESS STORY

SHE HAD THE GUTS TO LOSE HERS

Name: Linda Toomey

Age: 35

Height: 1.63 m/5'4"

Weight, Week 1: 66 kg/10 st 5 lb

Weight, Week 6: 57 kg/9 st

Body-Fat Percentage, Week 1: 35

Body-Fat Percentage, Week 6: 25

When Linda Toomey had her fourth baby, she knew that she had to get the weight off. She was still carrying an extra 9 kg/20 lb she'd gained from her third child, and she wanted to act quickly, because she knew the longer she waited, the harder it would be. At 66 kg/10 st 5 lb and with four children under the age of 6, she knew that her own health – and belly – might take a backseat to everything else going on in her life. 'I'm the queen of excuses,' she says.

Toomey also knew that she needed as much energy as possible – especially considering she wasn't getting a full night's sleep anyway, caring for a newborn.

after 12 months, they discovered that the low-fat eaters had not only gained back what they lost, but they had added an average of 2.75 kg/6 lb! The dieters who were allowed to eat fats, however, lost an average of 4 kg/9 lb – and kept it off.

So, as the song goes, Grease is the Word – as long as it's the right kind of grease. The two kinds of fats that you'll incorporate into your eating plan are polyunsaturated and monounsaturated. Polyunsaturated fats include the famous omega-3s, which are found in fish like salmon and tuna and work to help clear your

'At night, I expected to be tired,' she says. 'But I was tired 2 hours after I woke up.'

Her goals: get her body back, have more energy and strengthen her back to be able to meet the demands of carrying larger-than-average children.

'I tried other diets, but being so crazy and busy, I didn't have a lot of time for exercise or food preparation. I needed something that was easy and fast to prepare,' Toomey says.

She found it in the Abs Diet. 'It's not really a diet,' she says. 'It's a life-long eating plan. I think knowing that you can eat carbs and not resist cravings was one of the key factors. The eating plan was extremely easy to follow, and the whole family could enjoy the meals. I didn't have to prepare different foods for myself.'

Toomey also included the 20-minute exercise plan and strengthened her abdominals and lower back to the point where she has no problem lifting her children.

In 6 weeks, Toomey dropped 9 kg/20 lb and went from 35-per cent body fat to 25. And she also went from a size 16 dress to size 10.

'I'm hoping it motivates a lot of women,' Toomey says. 'In the past after being pregnant, the waist was extremely hard for me. I may have lost centimetres from everywhere else in the past, but the waist was my real difficult area. It's amazing how it progressed in a short time.'

arteries. More research shows that polyunsaturated fat also plays a role in helping speed your metabolism. Studies have shown that people who take omega-3s burned more calories throughout the day than those who don't. And a recent study of more than 35,000 women discovered that those who ate fish high in omega-3s had the lowest body mass indexes (BMIs) – even lower than vegetarians. (And if you're a vegetarian, there's still no excuse: flaxseed and flaxseed oil are loaded with omega-3s, and you can find them in health food shops. Get the ground flaxseed so you can toss it on cereal or into smoothies.)

The other kind of good fat – monounsaturated – is found in nuts, olives, avocados and olive and rapeseed (canola) oils. Monounsaturated fats reduce cholesterol levels as well, and they also help burn fat and keep you satiated. One study found that subjects who ate a meal with oil high in monounsaturated fats felt fuller than those who ate one cooked with the polyunsaturated kind. And that's a primary approach to how you need to eat: balance your foods with the ingredients that keep your hunger in check. You want to keep your stomach satisfied – not the people at Big & Tall.

The Appetite Suppressor: Fibre-Rich Carbohydrates

As I stated earlier in this chapter, it's not the 'carbohydrate' part you should be concerned about, it's the fibre part. Wholegrain breads and cereals, oats and berries – these are the real weapons of mass destruction, and the mass they seek to destroy is the one collecting around your waist.

There are two types of fibre: soluble and insoluble. Let's see if I can define them both in one paragraph without making you nod off.

Soluble fibre, like the kind you find in oats, apples and other fruits and grains, likes to hang out in your stomach. While it's hanging out, it does two things. Firstly, it slows digestion, giving you longer-burning energy throughout the day. Secondly, it bonds with digestive acids, which happen to be made from cholesterol. When fibre splits, it takes the digestive acids with it, forcing your body to pull cholesterol from your bloodstream to make more. Presto, your cholesterol profile improves. Insoluble fibre, meanwhile, does not like to hang around. It shoots through your plumbing like Dyno-Rod, picking up miscellaneous fats and whatever else happens to be loitering in your system and ushering them out the back. So both types of fibre help keep all your pipes and fittings in order and, if you eat them regularly, they should delay any need for professional plumbing services in the near future.

The Weight-Loss Wonder: Calcium

In the past few years, researchers have begun studying the effects of calcium-rich dairy foods on weight management. And quite frankly, it's hard not to be wowed by the evidence.

For example, researchers at Harvard Medical School showed that those who ate three servings of dairy foods a day – to total the recommended 1,200 milligrams of calcium daily – were 60 per cent less likely to be overweight. But some of the most exciting research came from a study in which researchers put subjects on diets that were 500 calories a day less than what they were used to eating. The subjects lost weight – about 455 g/1 lb of fat a week. But when researchers put another set of subjects on the same diet but added dairy to their meals, their fat loss doubled, to 900 g/2 lb a week. Same calorie intake, double the fat loss. Calcium, it seems, is going to be one of the most exciting new areas of research about weight loss and metabolism, and that's why it's an important part of the ABS DIET POWER 12.

Chapter 2

NEVER GO HUNGRY AGAIN

The ABS DIET POWER 12

GOVERNMENTS USE acronyms: CIA, MI5, EU. Media corporations use acronyms: ABC, BBC, CNN. We love acronyms because they're easy to remember. (Do you even recall what BBC stands for after all these years?)

The Abs Diet comes with its own acronym – the ABS DIET POWER 12. They are 12 foods you want to look for and fit into your eating plan whenever you can.

I don't know about you, but if I had to consult a chart, formulate some kind of substitution plan, or calculate calories at every turn, I'd starve. Eating plans need to be simple, because life is complicated. And that's what the ABS DIET POWER 12 is – simple. Figuratively, it stands for the principles of what this body-transforming diet is all about. Literally, it stands for:

Almonds and other nuts
Beans and pulses
Spinach and other green vegetables

Dairy (fat-free or low-fat milk, yogurt, cheese)
Instant and quick-cooking oats (unsweetened, unflavoured)
Eggs
Turkey, other lean meats and fish

Peanut butter
Olive oil
Wholegrain breads and cereals
Extra-protein (whey) powder
Raspberries and other berries

As you can see, these 12 foods, or food groups, if you will, constitute a veritable cornucopia of dietary choices. You can use the acronym when you're shopping, when you're cooking at home and when you're eating out.

The crux of the diet and *The Abs Diet Eat Right Every Time Guide* is that if you can revolve your meals around these 12 Powerfoods, you'll know exactly what to order, what to shop for and how to eat right every time. You'll have armed yourself with the 'friend' category of nutrients that will help your body lose fat and gain lean muscle, and you'll have shunned the 'enemy' category of junk foods that threaten to lay waste to your waist. Here's a quick overview of the ABS DIET POWER 12 and what they have to offer.

How to read the key: For at-a-glance scanning, I've included the following icons under the descriptions of each of the Abs Diet Powerfoods. Each icon demonstrates which important roles each food can help play in maintaining optimum health.

Builds muscle: Foods rich in muscle-building plant and animal proteins qualify for this seal of approval, as do foods rich in certain minerals linked to proper muscle maintenance, such as magnesium.

Helps prevent weight gain: Foods high in calcium and fibre (both of which protect against obesity), as well as foods that help build fat-busting muscle tissue, earn this badge of respect.

Strengthens bone: Calcium and vitamin D are the most important bone builders, and they protect the body against osteoporosis. But beware: high levels of sodium can leach calcium out of bone tissue. Fortunately, all of the Powerfoods are naturally low in sodium.

Lowers blood pressure: Any food that's not high in sodium can help lower blood pressure – and earn this designation – if it has beneficial amounts of potassium, magnesium or calcium.

Fights cancer: Research has shown that there is a lower risk of some types of cancer among people who maintain low-fat, high-fibre diets. You can also help foil cancer by eating foods that are high in calcium, beta-carotene or vitamin C. In addition, all cruciferous (cabbage-type) and allium (onion-type) vegetables get the cancer protection symbol because research has shown they help prevent certain kinds of cancer.

Improves immune function: Vitamins A, E, B_6 and C; folic acid; and the mineral zinc help to increase the body's immunity to certain types of disease. This icon indicates a Powerfood with high levels of one or more of these nutrients.

Fights heart disease: Artery-clogging cholesterol can lead to trouble if you eat foods that are predominant in saturated and trans fats, while foods that are high in monounsaturated or polyunsaturated fats will actually help protect your heart by keeping your cholesterol levels in check.

1: Almonds and Other Nuts

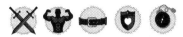

Superpowers: builds muscle, fights cravings

Secret weapons: protein, monounsaturated fats, vitamin E, fibre, magnesium, folic acid (peanuts), phosphorus

Fights against: obesity, heart disease, muscle loss, wrinkles, cancer, high blood pressure

Sidekicks: flaxseed, pumpkin seeds, sunflower seeds, avocados

Imposters: salted or smoked nuts

These days, you hear about good fats and bad fats the way you hear about good cops and bad cops. One's on your side, and one's gonna beat you silly. Biscuits fall into the latter category, but nuts are clearly out to help you. They contain the monounsaturated fats that clear your arteries and help you feel full.

All nuts are high in protein and monounsaturated fat. But almonds are like Jack Nicholson in *One Flew over the Cuckoo's Nest*: they're the king of the nuts. A handful of almonds provides half the amount of vitamin E you need in a day and 8 per cent of the calcium. Almonds also contain 19 per cent of your daily requirement of magnesium – a key component for muscle building. In a Western Washington University study, people taking extra magnesium were able to lift 20 per cent more weight and build more muscle than those who weren't. Eat as much as two handfuls of almonds a day. A Toronto University study found that men can eat this amount daily without gaining any extra weight. A study at Purdue University, Indiana, showed that people who ate nuts high in monounsaturated fat felt full an hour and a half longer than those who ate fat-free food (rice cakes, in this instance). If you eat 60 g/2 oz of almonds (about 24 of them), it should be enough to suppress your appetite – especially if you wash them down with 240 ml/8 fl oz of water. The fluid helps expand the fibre in the nuts to help you feel fuller. Also, eat almonds with the nuts' nutrient-rich skins on them.

Here are ways to seamlessly introduce almonds and other nuts into your diet.

▶ Add chopped nuts to peanut butter.

▶ Toss a handful of nuts on cereal, yogurt or ice cream.

SMART SUPPLEMENTS

You can get nearly every nutrient in the ABS DIET POWER 12 from a bottle or a can. Health food shops are filled with multivitamins and dietary supplements that promise better health and nutrition. But I want you to be eating real, wholesome, delicious foods, not popping pills.

One main reason – besides the fact that eating your meals in pill form makes you feel like you're on the set of *Logan's Run* – is that fruits, vegetables, whole grains and other Powerfoods offer not only the aforementioned vitamins, minerals and fibre, but hundreds of 'micronutrients', as well. These micronutrients – many of which are only now being studied and classified – may have tremendous protective properties that scientists are still trying to discover. So the more real food you eat, the more real nutrition you get.

That said, there are two nutrients that aren't readily available through traditional food sources. If you want to supplement your healthy diet with some extra weight-loss power, consider:

▶ Conjugated linoleic acid (CLA) is a fatty acid that's been shown to aid in weight loss. Researchers recently reported that subjects taking CLA for 1 year lost up to 8.7 per cent of their body fat. The recommended dosage is 3 grams daily.

▶ Pyruvate is an antioxidant that may help aid weight loss. In two trials, people taking pyruvate in addition to a low-fat diet stepped up their weight loss. The recommended dosage is 25 grams daily.

▶ Put almond slivers in an omelette.

▶ For a quick popcorn alternative, spray a handful of almonds with non-stick cooking spray and bake at 200° C/ 400° F/ gas 6 for 5 to 10 minutes. Take them out of the oven and sprinkle them with a mixture of either brown sugar and cinnamon or cayenne pepper and thyme.

One caveat, before you get all nutty: smoked and salted nuts don't make the cut here, because of their high sodium content. High sodium can mean high blood pressure.

Although it's not technically a nut, I want you to consider adding ground flaxseed to your food. One tablespoon contains only 60 calories, but it packs in omega-3 fatty acids and has nearly 4 grams of fibre. It has a nutty flavour, so you can sprinkle it into a lot of different recipes: add some to your meat or beans, spoon it over cereal or add a tablespoon to a smoothie.

2: Beans and Pulses

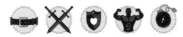

Superpowers: builds muscle, helps burn fat, regulates digestion

Secret weapons: fibre, protein, iron, folic acid

Fights against: obesity, colon cancer, heart disease, high blood pressure

Sidekicks: lentils, peas, bean dips, hummus, edamame (green soya beans)

Imposters: refried beans, which are high in saturated fats; baked beans, which are high in sugar

Most of us can trace our resistance to beans to some unfortunately timed intestinal upheaval (third-year maths class, a first date gone awry). But beans are, as the song says, good for your heart; the more you eat them, the more you'll be able to control your hunger. Black, butter, kidney, chickpea – you pick the bean (as long as it's not refried – refried beans are loaded with fat). Beans are a low-calorie food packed with protein, fibre and iron – ingredients crucial for building muscle and losing weight. Gastrointestinal disadvantages notwithstanding, beans serve as one of the key members of the Abs Diet cabinet because of all their nutritional power. In fact, you can swap a bean-heavy dish for a meat-heavy dish a couple of times per week; you'll be lopping a lot of saturated fat out of your diet and replacing it with higher amounts of fibre.

The best beans for your diet are:

▶ Soya beans

▶ Chickpeas

▶ Haricot beans

▶ Black beans

▶ Cannellini beans

▶ Kidney beans

▶ Butter beans

3: Spinach and Other Green Vegetables

Superpower: neutralizes free radicals, which are molecules that accelerate the ageing process

Secret weapons: vitamins including A, C and K; folic acid; minerals including calcium and magnesium; fibre; beta-carotene

Fights against: cancer, heart disease, stroke, obesity, osteoporosis

Sidekicks: cruciferous vegetables like broccoli and Brussels sprouts; green, yellow, red and orange vegetables like asparagus, beans and peppers (capsicums)

Imposters: none, as long as you don't fry them or smother them in fatty cheeses

You know vegetables are packed with important nutrients, but they're also a critical part of your body-changing diet. I like spinach in particular because one serving supplies nearly a full day's worth of vitamin A and half of your vitamin C. It's also loaded with folic acid – a vitamin that protects against heart disease, stroke and colon cancer. To incorporate spinach into your diet, you can take the fresh stuff and use it as lettuce on a sandwich or try stir-frying it with a little olive oil and garlic.

Another potent power vegetable is broccoli. It's high in fibre and more densely packed with vitamins and minerals than almost any other food. For instance, broccoli contains nearly 90 per cent of the vitamin C of fresh orange juice and almost half as much calcium as milk. It is also a powerful defender against diseases like cancer because it increases the enzymes that help detoxify carcinogens. Tip: with broccoli, you can skip the stalks. The florets have three times as much beta-carotene as the stems, and they're also a great source of other antioxidants. Sauté in olive oil and garlic and douse them with hot chilli sauce.

If you hate vegetables, you can learn to hide them but still reap the benefits. Try puréeing them and adding them to pasta sauces or chilli con carne. The more you chop and purée vegetables, the more invisible they become, and the easier it is for your body to absorb them.

4: Dairy (Fat-Free or Low-Fat Milk, Yogurt, Cheese)

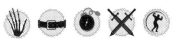

Superpowers: builds strong bones, fires up weight loss

Secret weapons: calcium, vitamins A and B_{12}, riboflavin, phosphorus, potassium

Fights against: osteoporosis, obesity, high blood pressure, cancer

Sidekicks: cottage cheese, low-fat soured cream

Imposters: whole milk, frozen yogurt

Dairy is nutrition's version of a typecast actor. It gets so much attention for one thing it does well – strengthening bones – that it gets little or no attention for all the other stuff it does well. It's about time for dairy to accept a breakout role as a vehicle for weight loss. Just take a look at the mounting evidence: a University of Tennessee study found that dieters who consumed between 1,200 and 1,300 milligrams of calcium a day lost nearly twice as much weight as dieters getting less calcium. In a study of 54 people at Purdue University, Indiana, those who took in 1,000 milligrams of calcium a day (about 700 ml/1¼ pints of skimmed milk) gained less weight over 2 years than those with low-calcium diets. Researchers think that calcium probably prevents weight gain by increasing the breakdown of body fat and hampering its formation. Low-fat yogurt, cheeses and other dairy products can play an important role in your diet. But as your major source of calcium, I recommend milk for one primary reason: volume. Liquids can take up valuable room in your stomach and send the signal to your brain that you're full. Adding in a sprinkling of chocolate powder can help curb sweet cravings while still providing nutritional power.

5: Instant and Quick-Cooking Oats (Unsweetened, Unflavoured)

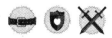

Superpowers: boosts energy and sex drive, reduces cholesterol, maintains blood sugar levels

Secret weapons: complex carbohydrates and fibre

Fights against: heart disease, diabetes, colon cancer, obesity

Sidekicks: high-fibre cereals like All-Bran

Imposters: cereals with added sugar and high-fructose corn syrup

Oatmeal is the Bo Derek of your larder: it's a perfect 10. You can eat it at breakfast to propel you through sluggish mornings, a couple of hours before a workout to feel fully energized by the time you hit the weights, or at night to avoid a late-night binge. I recommend instant or quick-cooking oats for convenience. But I want you to buy the unsweetened, unflavoured variety and use other Powerfoods such as milk and berries to enhance the taste. Preflavoured oats often come loaded with sugar calories.

Oats contain soluble fibre, meaning that it attracts fluid and stays in your stomach longer than insoluble fibre (the kind found in whole grains such as wheat and barley). Soluble fibre is thought to reduce blood cholesterol by binding with digestive acids made from cholesterol and sending them out of your body. When this happens, your liver has to pull cholesterol from your blood to make more digestive acids, and your bad cholesterol levels drop.

Trust me: you need more fibre, both soluble and insoluble. Doctors recommend we get between 18 and 25 grams of fibre per day, but many of us get half that. Fibre is like a bouncer for your body, kicking out troublemakers and showing them the door. Fibre protects you from heart disease, and it also protects you from colon cancer by sweeping carcinogens out of the intestines quickly.

A Penn State study also showed that oats sustain your blood sugar levels longer than many other foods, which keeps your insulin levels stable and ensures you won't be ravenous for the few hours that follow. That's good, because spikes in the production of insulin slow your metabolism and send a signal to the body that it's time to start storing fat. Since oats break down slowly in the stomach, they cause less of a spike in insulin levels than foods like bagels. Include oats in a smoothie or as your breakfast. (A US Navy study showed that simply eating breakfast raised metabolism by 10 per cent.)

Another cool fact about oats: preliminary studies indicate that oats raise the levels of free testosterone in your body, enhancing your body's ability to build muscle and burn fat and boosting your sex drive.

6: Eggs

Superpowers: builds muscle, burns fat

Secret weapons: protein, vitamin B_{12}, vitamin A

Fights against: obesity

Sidekicks: none

Imposters: none

For a long time, eggs were considered pure evil, and doctors were more likely to recommend tossing eggs at passing cars than into omelette pans. That's because just two eggs contain enough cholesterol to put you over your daily recommended intake. Though you can cut out some of the cholesterol by removing part of the yolk and using the whites, more and more research shows that eating an egg or two a day will not raise your cholesterol levels, as once previously believed. In fact, we've learned that most blood cholesterol is made by the body from dietary fat, not dietary cholesterol. And that's why you should take advantage of eggs and their powerful make-up of protein.

The protein found in eggs has the highest 'biological value' of protein – a measure of how well it supports your body's protein need – of any food. In other words, the protein in eggs is more effective in building muscle than protein from other sources, even milk and beef. Eggs also contain vitamin B_{12}, which is necessary for fat breakdown.

7: Turkey, Other Lean Meats and Fish

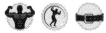

Superpowers: builds muscle, improves the immune system

Secret weapons: protein, iron, zinc, creatine (beef), omega-3 fatty acids (oily fish), vitamins B_6 (chicken and fish) and B_{12}, phosphorus, potassium

Fights against: obesity, various diseases

Sidekicks: shellfish, back bacon

Imposters: sausage, streaky bacon, cured meats, ham, fatty cuts of steak like T-bone and rib-eye

A classic muscle-building nutrient, protein is the base of any solid diet plan. You already know that it takes more energy for your body to digest the protein in meat than it does to digest carbohydrates or fat. Many studies support the notion that high-protein diets promote weight loss. In one study, researchers in Denmark found that men who substituted protein for 20 per cent of their carbs were able to increase their metabolism and increase the number of calories they burned every day by up to 5 per cent.

Among meats, turkey is a rare bird. Turkey breast is one of the leanest meats you'll find, and it packs nearly one-third of your daily requirements of niacin and vitamin B_6. The dark meat, if you prefer it, has lots of zinc and iron. One caution, though: if you're roasting a whole turkey for a family feast, avoid self-basting birds, which have been injected with fat.

Beef is another classic muscle-building protein food. It's the top food source for creatine – the substance your body uses when you lift weights. Beef does have a downside; it contains saturated fats, but some cuts have more than others. Look for topside, rump or fillet steak; sirloins are less fatty than prime ribs and T-bones. Wash down that steak with a glass of skimmed milk. Research shows that calcium (that magic bullet again!) may reduce the amount of saturated fat your body absorbs. Choose cuts on the left side of the chart below. They contain less fat but still pack high amounts of protein.

LEAN BEEF (55 calories and 2–3 grams of fat per 30-g/1-oz serving)	MEDIUM-FAT BEEF (75 calories and 5 grams of fat per 30-g/1-oz serving)
Fillet steak	Chuck steak
Minced beef (extra-lean or lean)	Corned beef
Roast beef	Minced beef (not labelled lean or extra-lean)
Skirt (flank) steak	

To cut down on saturated fats even more, concentrate on fish like tuna and salmon, because they contain a healthy dose of omega-3 fatty acids as well as protein. Those fatty acids lower levels of a hormone called leptin in your body. Several recent studies suggest that leptin directly influences your metabolism: the higher your leptin levels, the more readily your body stores calories as fat. Researchers at the University of Wisconsin found that mice with low leptin levels have faster metabolisms and are able to burn fat faster than animals with higher leptin levels. Mayo Clinic researchers studying the diets of two African tribes found that the tribe that ate fish frequently had leptin levels nearly five times lower than the tribe that primarily ate vegetables. A bonus benefit: researchers in Stockholm studied the diets of more than 6,000 men and found that those who ate no fish had three times the risk of prostate cancer than those who ate it regularly. It's the omega-3s that inhibit prostate cancer growth.

8: Peanut Butter

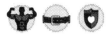

Superpowers: boosts testosterone, builds muscle, burns fat

Secret weapons: protein, monounsaturated fat, vitamin E, niacin, magnesium

Fights against: obesity, muscle loss, wrinkles, cardiovascular disease

Sidekicks: cashew and almond butters

Imposters: mass-produced sugary and trans fatty peanut butters

Yes, PB has its disadvantages: it's high in calories, and it doesn't go down well when you order it in three-star restaurants. But it's packed with those heart-healthy monounsaturated fats that can increase your body's production of testosterone, which can help your muscles grow and your fat melt. In one 18-month-long experiment, people who integrated peanut butter into their diets maintained weight loss better than those on low-fat plans. A recent study from the University of Illinois showed that diners who had monounsaturated fats before a meal (in this case, it was olive oil) ate 25 per cent fewer calories during that meal than those who didn't.

Practically speaking, PB also works because it's a quick and versatile snack, and it tastes good. Since a diet that includes an indulgence like peanut butter doesn't leave you feeling deprived, it's easier to follow and won't make you fall prey to other cravings. Use it on an apple, on the go, or to add flavour to potentially bland smoothies. Two caveats: you can't gorge on it because of its fat content; limit yourself to about 3 tablespoons per day. And you should look for all-natural peanut butter, not the mass-produced brands that have added sugar and trans fat.

9: Olive Oil

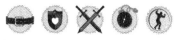

Superpowers: lowers cholesterol and boosts the immune system

Secret weapons: monounsaturated fat, vitamin E

Fights against: obesity, cancer, heart disease, high blood pressure

Sidekicks: rapeseed (canola) oil, peanut oil, sesame oil

Imposters: vegetable and hydrogenated vegetable oils, trans fatty acids, margarine and reduced-fat spreads

You read extensive information on the value of high-quality fats like olive oil in Chapter 1. But it's worth reiterating here: olive oil and its brethren will help you eat less by controlling your food cravings; they'll also help you burn fat and keep your cholesterol in check. Do you need any more reason to pass the bottle?

10: Wholegrain Breads and Cereals

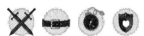

Superpower: prevents your body from storing fat

Secret weapons: fibre, protein, thiamin, riboflavin, niacin, pyridoxine, vitamin E, magnesium, zinc, potassium, iron, calcium

Fights against: obesity, cancer, high blood pressure, heart disease

Sidekicks: brown rice, wholewheat pastas

Imposters: processed bakery products like white bread, bagels and doughnuts; breads labelled wheat rather than wholewheat

There's only so long a person can survive on an all-protein diet or an all-salad diet or an all-anything diet. You will crave carbohydrates because your body needs carbohydrates. The key is to eat the ones that have been the least processed – carbs that still have all their heart-healthy, tummy-busting fibre intact.

Grains like wheat, corn, oats, barley and rye are seeds that come from grasses, and they're broken into three parts – the germ, the bran and the endosperm. Think of a kernel of corn (maize). The biggest part of the kernel – the part that blows up when you make popcorn – is the endosperm. Nutritionally it's pretty much a big dud. It contains starch, a little protein and some B vitamins. The germ is the smallest part of the grain; in a sweetcorn kernel, it's that little white seed-like thing. But while it's small, it packs the most nutritional power. It contains protein, oils and the B vitamins thiamin, riboflavin, niacin and pyridoxine. It also has vitamin E and the minerals magnesium, zinc, potassium and iron. The bran is the third part of the grain and the part where all the fibre is stored. It's a coating around the endosperm that contains B vitamins, zinc, calcium, potassium, magnesium and other minerals.

So what's the point of this little biology lesson? Well, get this: when food manufacturers process and refine grains, guess which two parts get tossed out? Yup, the bran, where all the fibre and minerals are, and the germ, where all the protein and vitamins are. And what they keep – the nutritionally bankrupt endosperm (that is, starch) – gets made into pasta, white rice, bagels, white bread and just about every other wheat product and baked good you'll find. Crazy, right? But if you eat products made with all the parts of the grain – wholegrain bread, wholewheat pasta, brown rice – you get all the nutrition that food manufacturers are otherwise trying to cheat you out of.

Wholegrain carbohydrates can play an important role in a healthy lifestyle. In an 11-year study of 16,000 middle-aged people, researchers at the University of Minnesota found that consuming three daily servings of whole grains can reduce a person's mortality risk over the course of a decade by 23 per cent. (Tell that to your friend who's eating low-carb.) Wholegrain bread keeps insulin levels low, which keeps you from storing fat. In this diet, it's especially versatile because it'll supplement any kind of meal with little prep time. Toast for breakfast, sandwiches for lunch, bread with a dab of peanut butter for a snack. Don't believe the hype. Carbs – the right kind of carbs – are good for you.

Warning: food manufacturers are very sneaky. Sometimes,

CAN YOU STOMACH THIS?

When I tell people about the Abs Diet, I'm often asked about the issue of portion control. In most diets, portion control is a key element, but the Abs Diet comes with its own portion control built in. Because you'll be eating lots of fibre, protein and healthy fats, the foods you eat on the Abs Diet will fill you up and give you long-running energy, so you won't feel the need to binge and won't have the urge to stuff your stomach like Santa's sack. But just for kicks, let's look at what happens to your body when you do overeat.

▶ Your stomach, which is the size of your closed fist, doesn't crave more servings. When you're full, it is, too.

▶ But if you're eating very quickly – a common problem with junk food – your stomach becomes distended and can swell to as much as three times its original size. It then pushes against your lungs and diaphragm.

▶ If you really overeat, some of the food may not immediately reach your stomach, so it loiters in your oesophagus, causing acid reflux-related belching and nausea.

▶ Your liver works overtime to digest the surplus food by producing excess bile – an emulsifier that helps fats and oils pass through your intestines. Your intestines also crank out extra digestive enzymes.

▶ After all this stressful work, your gastrointestinal system can't take it and rebels. Your body looks for a way to dump the excess cargo – by any means necessary.

after refining away all the vitamins, fibre and minerals from wheat, they'll claim to 'put back the goodness' by adding wheat-germ. It's a trick! Truly nutritious breads and other products will say wholewheat or wholegrain. Don't be fooled.

11: Extra-Protein (Whey) Powder

Superpowers: builds muscle, burns fat

Secret weapons: protein, cysteine, glutathione

Fights against: obesity

Sidekick: ricotta cheese

Imposter: soya protein

Protein powder? What the heck is that? It's the only Abs Diet Powerfood that you may not be able to find at the supermarket, but it's the one that's worth the trip to a health food shop. I'm talking about powdered whey protein, a type of animal protein that packs a muscle-building wallop. If you add whey powder to your meal – in a smoothie, for instance – you may very well have created the most powerful fat-burning meal possible. Whey protein is a high-quality protein that contains essential amino acids that build muscle and burn fat. But it's especially effective because it has the highest amount of protein for the fewest number of calories, making it fat's kryptonite. Smoothies with some whey powder can be most effective before a workout. A 2001 study at the University of Texas found that weightlifters who drank a shake containing amino acids and carbohydrates before working out increased their protein synthesis (their ability to build muscle) more than lifters who drank the same shake after exercising. Since exercise increases bloodflow to tissues, the theory goes that having whey protein in your system when you work out may lead to a greater uptake of amino acids – the building blocks of muscle – in your muscle.

But that's not all. Whey protein can help protect your body against prostate cancer. Whey is a good source of cysteine, which your body uses to build a prostate cancer-fighting antioxidant called glutathione. Adding just a small amount may increase glutathione levels in your body by up to 60 per cent.

By the way, the one great source of whey protein in your supermarket is ricotta cheese. Unlike other cheeses, which are made from milk curds, ricotta is made from whey – a good reason to visit your local Italian restaurant.

12: Raspberries and Other Berries

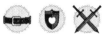

Superpowers: protects your heart; enhances eyesight; improves balance, coordination and short-term memory; prevents cravings

Secret weapons: antioxidants, fibre, vitamin C, tannins (cranberries)

Fights against: heart disease, cancer, obesity

Sidekicks: most other fruits, especially apples and grapefruit

Imposters: jams, most of which eliminate fibre and add sugar

Depending on your taste, any berry will do. I like raspberries as much for their power as for their taste. They carry powerful levels of antioxidants, all-purpose compounds that help your body fight heart disease and cancer. The berries' flavonoids may also help your eyesight, balance, coordination and short-term memory. A bowl (145 g/5 oz) of raspberries packs 4 grams of fibre and more than 100 per cent of your daily requirement of vitamin C.

Blueberries are also loaded with the soluble fibre that, like oats, keeps you fuller longer. In fact, they're one of the most healthy foods you can eat. Blueberries beat 39 other fruits and vegetables in the antioxidant power ratings. (One study also found that rats that ate blueberries were more coordinated and smarter than rats that didn't.)

Strawberries contain another valuable form of fibre called pectin (as do grapefruit, peaches, apples and oranges). In a study from the *Journal of the American College of Nutrition*, subjects drank plain orange juice or juice spiked with pectin. The people who got the loaded juice felt fuller after drinking it than those who got the juice without the pectin. The difference lasted for an impressive 4 hours.

MIDNIGHT MADNESS

If you're dying for a midnight snack, chances are you're probably more bored, restless or worried than you are hungry – especially if you've eaten six meals already today. The key here is to do as little harm as possible and to get back to bed. Milk, oats and bananas contain trace amounts of melatonin, the send-me-to-sleep hormone. Combine them all in one bowl (one instant oats packet made with milk and topped with half a sliced banana) or just have one alone. Back-ups: a small bowl (30 g/1 oz or so) of wholegrain cereal with milk, 2 fig rolls, or 60 ml/2 fl oz ice cream.

The Abs Diet Bull's Eye

Variety being the spice of life and all, you're often going to have the opportunity and the desire to mix in foods that don't fall squarely into the ABS DIET POWER 12. That's fine, as long as you keep your eye on the target and try to mix at least two Powerfoods into each meal and snack.

To help keep you focused on the ABS DIET POWER 12, I've created a little game I call the Abs Diet Bull's Eye. In the centre of this chart are the foods you want to concentrate on. Around them, in concentric layers, are additional foods you'll no doubt run across every day.

Eat Rarely

Bagels · Baked goods, such as cake and biscuits · Beef, fatty cuts such as T-bone · Beer, regular · Breads, white flour · Duck · Jellies · Pasta, with creamy sauce · Pastries · Ribs · Soft drinks · Soup, creamy · Vegetables, creamed or fried · Bacon · Gravy · Refried beans

Eat Occasionally

Apple sauce · Baked beans · Baked potatoes · Beer, light · Butter, light · Chocolate · Coffee, with skimmed milk · Lamb · Lasagne · Macaroni · Margarine, trans fat-free · Nuts, salted or smoked

Eat Often

Apples · Asparagus · Avocados · Back bacon · Bananas · Brown rice · Citrus fruits and juices · Fruit juice, no sugar added · Game lean choices such as venison, ostrich · Garlic · Lentils · Melons · Mushrooms · Peaches · Peanut/groundnut oil · Peas · Peppers (capsicums) · pizza, plain or with vegetables · Popcorn, fat-free · Rapeseed/canola oil · Shellfish, steamed · Soup, stock-based or baked · Sunflower seeds · Sweet potatoes

ABS DIET

Almonds
  and other nuts
Beans and
  other pulses
Spinach
  and other green
  vegetables
Dairy
  (fat-free or low-fat)
Instant oats
Eggs
Turkey, other
  lean meats (lean
  steak, chicken) and
  fish

Indulge in them from time to time, but try to stay as focused on the centre of the bull's eye as you can. You have the flexibility to eat what you want, but this bull's eye will help you focus on the centre goal. The closer you stick to the inside, the healthier your diet will be and the better results you'll see. And if your dinner-time darts are always hitting outside the ring, then I think you may need to re-evaluate your form.

POWERFOODS

Peanut butter
Olive oil
Wholegrain
  breads and cereal
Extra-protein
  (whey) powder
Raspberries
  and other berries

Eat Often

Tomatoes · Tomato sauce · Vegetable juice · Veggie burgers · Wine, red · Tea · Tofu · Flaxseed · Sweetcorn · Edamame (green soya beans) · Yogurt, frozen · Wine, white · Veal · Sorbet · Pasta, wholewheat with tomato sauce and/or vegetables · Salsa · Sesame oil · Onions · Ricotta cheese · Prunes · Pumpkin seeds · Cruciferous vegetables, such as broccoli and brussels sprouts · almond and cashew · Nut butters, such as · Fruit, dried · Aubergine (eggplant)

Eat Occasionally

Muesli, low-fat · Muesli or energy bars · Digestive biscuits · French fries, oven-baked · Pork, tenderloin/fillet · Rice, white · Sauerkraut · Jam or marmalade · Ham, lean · Honey · Ice cream, low-fat · Sweets

Eat Rarely

Burgers, fast food · Cereals, sugared · Pizza, frozen or with extra cheese and meat toppings · Chicken, fried · Chicken wings · Crisps (potato chips) · Dairy products, full-fat · Doughnuts · French fries · Salad dressing, creamy · Sausage, pork · Seafood, fried · Popcorn, buttered

HE BEAT THE CURSE OF THE FAMILY GUT

Name: Jim Phillips

Age: 37

Height: 1.86 m/6'1"

Weight, Week 1: 86 kg/13 st 8 lb

Weight, Week 6: 76.5 kg/12 st 1 lb

Body-Fat Percentage, Week 1: 24

Body-Fat Percentage, Week 6: 15

Ever since secondary school, Jim Phillips had been gaining weight – not all at once, but just a kilogram or so every year. At one point, he found himself at 98 kg/15 st 5 lb and decided he needed to do something about it. So he took up running, started cutting down on his fat intake, and concentrated on a more vegetarian-like diet. He lost weight and got down to 86 kg/13 st 8 lb. And he stayed at this weight – for 5 years. But still, Phillips's gut lingered on.

'I think I kinda wore the weight well, but I knew I was definitely overweight – even if other people didn't notice it,' he says.

One of the places Phillips wore his weight was the infamous Phillips family gut (which he'd inherited through years of fizzy drinks, pizza and bagels). After reaching that plateau of 86 kg/13 st 8 lb, Phillips resigned himself to the fact that he was going to stay there, especially as he got older.

Then, he found the Abs Diet.

'As soon as I saw the book, I really liked it because of the approach –
telling you the foods to eat, not what you can't,' Phillips says.
'Psychologically, that was one of the biggest things. I like feeling
good about what I'm eating.'

Phillips tried the Abs Diet – eating six times a day (up from his habit of
light meals early in the day and eating a big dinner) and following an
exercise programme that emphasizes strength-training and interval-
training as the means to burning fat. He really feels that his change in
exercise helped him. 'I was definitely into a lackadaisical routine the last
4 years. When I changed to a shorter routine and higher intensity, I
noticed the difference.'

The effect: he dropped 9.5 kg/21 lb in 6 weeks, 9 percentage points off
his body-fat percentage and 12 cm/4½ in off his waist. Plus, he has
much better energy and fitness levels. Though he ran regularly when he
was 86 kg/13 st 8 lb, he can really feel the difference now. 'I never felt
as good running as I feel now. My knees aren't hurting. Hills are so
much easier. I did 13 miles yesterday,' says Phillips, who has run
marathons and is training for another. 'Before, I wouldn't have been able
to walk the next day after doing that distance. Now it doesn't even
bother me.'

While he still indulges in an occasional doughnut, he's made a change –
for good. 'After the fifth or sixth week on the diet, it hit me that I really
didn't remember what my old habits were,' Phillips says. 'The new ways
just became natural and something I wanted to live with and how I
wanted to eat. It wasn't going to be something I fell off because I could
eat the foods I like to eat.'

Chapter 3

THE SIX STEPS TO LIFELONG LEANNESS

Guidelines for Easy Eating

LOTS OF GOOD THINGS come in sixes. Besides the Six Nations rugby and cans of beer, there's also that group of muscles that gets title billing on this book. And then there's the Abs Diet guidelines. Six of them. That's it.

It all goes back to the simple principle of, well, simplicity. No matter how nutritionally responsible popular diets are (some are and some aren't, by the way), most of them are more high maintenance than an old Fiat. They require you to do complicated maths, keep dietary journals, or stay 'in the zone' (wherever the heck that is). Well, forget that. Instead, I've eliminated all the complex elements and boiled the Abs Diet down to six simple guidelines that don't require a degree in home economics or exotic ingredients you need to order from Madagascar.

What you'll find are that these six general principles aren't really rules; they just serve as the map that shows you the way to your ultimate destination: a lean, strong and healthy body.

Guideline 1: Eat six meals a day

When people are introduced to the Abs Diet, their first question is this: 'How can I lose weight if I'm eating twice as many meals?' The explanation is simple – and delicious.

See, nature doesn't much care if you have abs, which is why Cro-Magnon man didn't look good in Speedos. Our bodies evolved to do one thing: stay alive long enough to pass our genes on to the next generation. When our ancestors roamed the jungles and plains, they encountered frequent times of deprivation and hardship. So just like bears in winter, our bodies became adept at storing calories, in the form of fat, to tide us over during times when food was scarce.

The more frequently the body is exposed to times of deprivation, the more it conspires to store fat and to jettison lean muscle tissue. That's because muscle requires more calories to maintain it than fat does. The drought hits, the herds move on, and our ancestor starts living on his own muscle tissue. When food returns, his body reacts by bulking up with fat so he can make it through future lean times.

Nowadays, the herd never moves on; it's always there, 24 hours a day, at the drive-through. But people who go on calorie-restrictive diets create a modern version of starvation: they're not eating enough calories to maintain their lean muscle tissue. (In fact, most diets are not fat-loss diets, they're muscle-loss diets.) And as soon as people go off their diets, boom: the body instinctively begins storing fat. It doesn't know that it's being starved on purpose; it only knows it needs to survive the next diet.

But there's more bad news for the starvation-diet set. By burning away muscle, they're sacrificing the body's greatest weapon in the fight against flab. As I said above, muscle requires many more calories to maintain it than fat does. In fact, for each 455 g/1 lb of muscle you gain, your body burns up to 50 extra calories a day, just sitting still. Now let's say you go on a restrictive diet for a week, and you lose 1.8 kg/4 lb, and half of that is muscle. When you end your diet and return to eating as you normally do, you may be taking in the same number of calories you once did – but your body actually requires 100 calories a day less, because of the muscle you lost. So where do those calories go? Right to your gut. It takes only 3,500 calories to build 455 g/1 lb of fat. So you've now programmed your

---

ABS DIET SUCCESS STORY

THE ABS DIET HEALS A BAD BACK

Name: Kyle Snay

Age: 36

Height: 1.98 m/6'5"

Weight, Week 1: 103 kg/16 st 3 lb

Weight, Week 6: 93 kg/14 st 9 lb

Weight, Week 9: 90 kg/14 st 3 lb

Kyle Snay knew he needed to get back into shape – fast. Motivation to get in shape came in droves.

Reason 1: His dad. Several years earlier, Snay had made plans to visit his father – whom he didn't know well because his parents had been divorced. But 6 months before Snay was to make his pilgrimage, his dad dropped dead of a heart attack. That's when it hit Snay that his health was something he needed better control of.

Reason 2: His kids. 'I was a walking biscuit barrel for years,' Snay says. 'When my wife was pregnant with our second child, I said that I really needed to do something to get back in shape at least for my family. I was trying to keep up with our 2 year old, and it was exhausting.'

Reason 3: His back. Snay, who's had a herniated disc for 10 years, says, 'My big flare-up came when I bent down to pick up a Doritos chip.' After years of twinges, spasms and pain that laid him up for a couple of days at a time, he was told by doctors his choices were surgery or physical therapy.

body to gain 455 g/1 lb of fat every 35 days – or more than 4.5 kg/ 10 lb in the coming year. Some diet plan, huh?

And yet this is the crux of yo-yo dieting, and it's one of the worst things you can do for your figure and your health. But here's the thing: most of us go on mini-starvation diets every single day. When we limit ourselves to three meals a day, we're asking our

Snay chose neither. He chose the Abs Diet.

After deciding he was going to lose weight, Snay went searching for something hassle-free. 'I didn't want to count calories or carbs or fat. I read about the Abs Diet in *Men's Health* and noticed results immediately.'

Before, Snay never paid attention to what he ate: his staple foods included ice cream and whole packets of chocolate biscuits. He immediately changed his diet and saw the weight fall off. Plus, he got a bonus out of it: a better back. 'Since I started, I haven't had a twinge, a spasm, or anything – nothing. My back is completely fine,' he says. 'It's just unreal. That was a huge plus that I wasn't even expecting.'

Snay says he really stuck to the principles but appreciates the diet's flexibility. Eating six times a day, he says, makes you feel like you're never really 'on a diet'.

Now, almost 14 kg/30 lb lighter, Snay retrained his metabolism – so much so that he lost his last 2.25 kg/5 lb even when he had to take a week off from exercise and sneak in a few extra cheat meals because he was away at a business conference. He also invents his own recipes following the ABS DIET POWER 12. 'I know people who are still trying to do Atkins, and they just pour meat into their stomach. In a couple of weeks, they're still walking around like a bowl of pudding because they're not doing any exercise, and they're taking too many shortcuts,' he says.

'I can't ever see myself going back to who I was before,' Snay says. 'I just can't wait until it gets warm again. I'm going to go out and wash my car – with my shirt off for the first time in years. I'll even stay out there longer and wash my neighbour's car, too.'

bodies to operate normally all the time, even though we're inter-mittently depriving it of fuel, then dumping big heaps of calories into it every 6 hours or so. That's why eating three square meals will make you round. But if you break those meals into six of them, you're getting a steady stream of fuel throughout the day to balance what your body is doing.

In fact, the new catchphrase in obesity science is 'energy bal-ance'. Energy balance refers to taking in throughout the day a similar number of calories as you're burning off. As long as you're constantly fuelling your body with small meals, you're constantly teaching it to shed fat. Ideally, you're trying to keep your hourly calorie surplus or deficit within 300 or 500 calories at all times, meaning that you're never going long periods without eating, and you're never overloading your system with too many calories at one sitting. As you burn calories throughout the day – by exercis-ing, by walking from the car park, by jumping up and down screaming, if that's your thing – the calories you ingest should stay within similar levels of the calories you burn. That's balance – never having too many calories and never being starved for more. In one study, researchers gave two sets of dieters the same daily calorie intake. But one group ate those calories in two big meals, while the other group ate them in six small meals spread throughout the day. At the end of the study, those who ate six meals a day lost an average of 5 kg/11 lb in two weeks; those who ate the same number of calories in just two meals a day also lost 5 kg/11 lb, but they lost 1.4 kg/3 lb more of muscle than men eat-ing 6 meals who lost 1.4 kg/3 lb more of fat.

So the Abs Diet works in two ways: by maintaining your energy balance and by helping you build new muscle. The more lean mus-cle mass you have, the more energy it takes to fuel it – meaning that calories go to your muscles to sustain them rather than being con-verted to fat. That's why I call muscle-building exercise the magic bullet in the chamber – the secret weapon in your fight against fat.

You'll read much more about the Abs Diet Workout in Chapter 11, and you'll learn how you can build new muscle that jump-starts your metabolism and turns your body into a fat-burning machine. In the meantime, I want you to keep this equation in mind:

MORE FOOD = MORE MUSCLE = LESS FLAB

The alternative:

LESS FOOD = LESS MUSCLE = MORE FLAB

Oh, and one more thing: if you eat six times a day, you never get hungry. If you never get hungry, you never get tired, cranky or miserable. And if you never get hungry, tired, cranky or miserable, you never feel the need to drown your hunger pangs or energy drain in an orgy of ice cream.

To keep the fat-burners firing, eat your six meals like this:

▶Alternate larger meals and smaller ones.

▶ Eat your snacks roughly 2 hours before lunch, 2 hours before dinner and roughly 2 hours after dinner.

▶Eat to fit your own schedule and lifestyle, but an ideal schedule would look something like this:

8 AM: Breakfast
11 AM: Snack
1 PM: Lunch
4 PM: Snack
6 PM: Dinner
8 PM: Snack

Guideline 2: Revolve your eating around the ABS DIET POWER 12

The ABS DIET POWER 12 is your ticket to eating better anywhere, anytime. While every meal won't consist entirely of Powerfoods, the more Powerfoods you can squeeze into your day, the more quickly and effectively you'll change your body and your life.

For example, let's say you're trapped in some nutritional equivalent of Dante's Inferno, where the only food you have to eat comes out of a vending machine. You could choose the Coke and the tortilla chips and a Kit Kat for dessert. Or you could peer through the glass and look for Powerfoods. They're in there . . . the fat-free popcorn, the unsalted peanuts, the low-fat chocolate milk.

Let's see . . . fizzy drinks, tortilla chips and Kit Kat, or chocolate milk, popcorn and peanuts. Both sound like junk-food meals, right? So which do you choose? Here's where the magic of the Powerfoods comes into play:

VENDING MACHINE MEAL 1:

Can of Coke 129 calories/554 kJ, 0 g protein, 25 g carbohydrates, 0 g fat, 0 g fibre, 25 mg sodium

45 g/1¹/₂ oz bag of nacho cheese tortilla chips 207 calories/ 867 kJ, 3 g protein, 27 g carbohydrates, 10 g fat (2 g saturated), 2.5 g fibre, 387 mg sodium

Kit Kat (4 fingers) 220 calories/924 kJ, 3 g protein, 28 g carbohydrates, 11 g fat (7 g saturated), 0 g fibre, 52 mg sodium

VENDING MACHINE MEAL 2:

240 ml/8 fl oz low-fat chocolate milk 150 calories/641 kJ, 9 g protein, 23 g carbohydrates, 2 g fat (2 g saturated), 0 g fibre, 108 mg sodium

Plain popcorn (30 g/1 oz) 178 calories/740 kJ, 2 g protein, 15 g carbohydrates, 12 g fat (1 g saturated), 1 g fibre, 1 mg sodium

30 g/1 oz bag of unsalted peanuts 169 calories/701 kJ, 8 g protein, 4 g carbohydrates, 14 g fat (2 g saturated), 2 g fibre, 1 mg sodium

What a difference choosing the Powerfoods can make: Meal 1 has about 50 more calories, and pales in comparison nutritionally to Meal 2. By making your choices based on the Powerfoods, you get three times as much protein and significantly less saturated fat and sodium.

And that's something you can do no matter where you are, because every supermarket, every restaurant, every vending machine and every movie-theatre concession stand offers something that contains one or more Powerfoods. And that, my friends, will keep you losing weight – without driving you nuts.

While you're negotiating the nutrition wasteland, I'd like you to keep these three thoughts in mind:

▶Incorporate two to three Powerfoods into each of your three major meals and at least one or two of them into each of your three snacks.

▶Diversify your food at every meal to make sure you have a combination of protein, carbohydrates and healthy fat.

▶Make sure you sneak a little bit of protein into each snack.

Guideline 3: Drink smoothies regularly

I'll never forget something that one of the first followers of the Abs Diet said. He lost some 9 kg/20 lb in the first 6 weeks, and he attributed most of that loss to one part of the diet: the smoothies.

See, smoothies are more than just faux milk shakes packed with healthy ingredients. They're one of the keys to the Abs Diet, because they pack your day with more energy than a busload of cheerleaders. In a recent study, researchers found that meal-replacement shakes work brilliantly as a weight-loss method. Subjects who replaced two daily meals with shakes or meal-replacement bars lost about 9 per cent of their original body weight.

More importantly, smoothies feature everything you could possibly want out of a food, like:

▶Ease: They take less than 3 minutes to make

▶Taste: Like dessert, with one exception. They're guilt-free.

▶Satisfaction: Because they're so thick and packed with Powerfoods, they take up valuable room in your stomach to keep you full for hours.

►Effectiveness: With the secret fat-fighter calcium, and satiating fibre and protein, they're some of the most potent meals or snacks you can make.

While Chapter 8 gives you recipes for 27 different kinds of smoothies, I'd also encourage you to mix and match ingredients that fit your tastes. That's the great thing about smoothies. All you have to know is how to open a lid and press a button to make one. So dump in whatever Powerfoods you like, whether it's berries, peanut butter or oats, and experiment with your own flavours (I advise against the salmon). Then follow these guidelines.

►Drink one or two 240-ml/8-fl oz smoothies a day, as a meal substitute or snack. In one study, researchers found that regularly drinking meal replacements increased a man's chance of losing weight and keeping it off for longer than a year.

►Add ice cubes and blend your smoothie for at least 3 minutes. Thicker shakes incorporate a little more air and water but have an increased satiating effect. In one study, researchers found that people stayed fuller longer when they drank thick drinks than when they drank thin ones. Another study found that men who drank yogurt shakes that had been blended until they doubled in volume ate 96 fewer calories a day than men who drank shakes of normal thickness.

►Don't skimp on the yogurt. A University of Tennessee study found that men who added three servings of yogurt a day to their diets lost 61 per cent more body fat and 81 per cent more stomach fat over 12 weeks than men who didn't eat yogurt. Calcium, baby!

Guideline 4: Stop counting

On the Abs Diet, you'll count the number of kg/lb you've lost, you'll count the notches on your belt you've gained, you may even count your lucky stars. But one thing you will not count is calories. Counting calories is for suckers.

For one, most people don't have the time or discipline to record every carrot stick they eat or weigh the three slices of turkey breast they carved. And two, all calories are not made equally when it comes to metabolism. Instead, the important thing is to eat the right foods. If you do, your body will essentially regulate your caloric intake all by itself. By including a good balance of fibre and protein, you'll be full throughout the day.

What you want to do is think about – not record – the amount of food you eat by sticking to one helping of each food group you eat and keeping the total contents of each meal contained to the diameter of your plate (and please, no high-rise mashed potatoes).

Guideline 5: Watch what you drink

I think a diet with lots of restrictions is like a roller-coaster without hills or a zoo without animals. What's the point of having a diet plan if it's so regimented and boring that nobody's going to be able to follow it? That's why the Abs Diet is about what you can eat, not what you can't. But the one place you really have to be careful is in what you drink.

Alcohol and fizzy drinks, along with a lot of juice blends, contain empty, non-nutritious calories that will work against you in pursuit of a better body. While alcohol has some health benefits in moderation, it also encourages you to eat more, slows down fat-burning and increases fat-storing. Drink water (eight 240 ml/ 8-fl oz glasses is ideal), diet drinks and skimmed milk. I encourage you to keep the booze in the cooler for the first 6 weeks of the plan, but if you drink, limit yourself to no more than two or three drinks a week.

Guideline 6: Go ahead, cheat

Most of us are rebels at heart – inside each of us lies an inner James Dean or Keith Richards, an Ali or a Madonna, someone who wants to break the rules and make the world march to their own tune. Well, rebellion is built right into the Abs Diet.

On the Abs Diet, I want you to cheat – with one whatever-you-want meal a week. That way, you can satisfy your cravings without derailing your commitment to the ABS DIET POWER 12. Of course, in the Abs Diet, there are enough great variations that you'll probably lose the urge for pizza, chocolate or chocolate-flavoured pizza pretty quickly. In fact, many people who've used the Abs Diet reported that they didn't even feel the urge to cheat, but they loved the fact that they had it as an option.

Now, if you're going to cheat on me, I want you to do it consci-entiously. When considering an adulterous encounter with an unhealthy food bear in mind the following:

▶Plan it. If you schedule your cheat meal, you'll be less likely to eat on impulse at other times during the week. Make it every Friday, when you meet the gang from work for a beer. Or every Sunday, when you treat yourself to cake and ice cream while watching a DVD.

▶Really, do it. While you don't have to cheat, it may help you in the long run. Researchers at the American National Institutes of Health found that men who ate twice as many calories in a day as normal increased their metabolism by 9 per cent in the 24-hour period that followed.

▶Stick to one a week. The cheat meal is like walking on a cliffside track. It's entirely safe – unless you step over the edge. You need to view the cheat meal as satisfaction instead of temptation and remain focused on your weight-loss goals. You'll be better off for it.

Chapter 4

SHOP 'TIL YOU DROP (WEIGHT)

The Complete Abs Diet Grocery List

AS FAR AS I'M CONCERNED, every time someone walks into a supermarket, they should play 'Welcome to the Jungle' over the loudspeaker. Supermarkets are some of the most confusing and mind-numbing places on earth. Supermarkets have one goal: to sell you more calories than you actually came in to buy. The easiest foods to find are usually the worst for you (a special on doughnuts!), and in the checkout lane, eight rows of chocolate taunt you like rival fans at a football match. There's a reason why they're called supermarkets, you know; they're super marketers.

So next time you go food shopping, you should notice things, like . . . the confectionery aisle never moves. Sure, the junk – and it usually is junk – at the end of each aisle may shift, but the basic layout never changes. You can use this to your advantage. Make a list before you go. Be specific; instead of writing 'snacks' and winding up with 5 different flavours of potato chips (crisps) in your trolley, write 'yogurt' or 'flaked almonds'. This way, you'll be able to make tactical strikes; quickly buy exactly what you need instead of the crap they're trying to foist off on you. Here's your guide to marching down the aisle in style.

Produce: Work the Greens

Most produce is just as nutritious frozen as it is fresh, so be judicious. If you use it up slowly, pack your freezer. If you burn through greens like Vijay Singh, stick with fresh (taste and texture will be better).

Fresh raspberries, blueberries and strawberries: Don't think you'll finish them in 3 to 5 days? Buy frozen instead.

Bananas: Avoid too-green ones. They'll add a strange tang to a smoothie.

Lemons, limes, oranges, grapefruit: Pick fruits that feel heavy; it means they have more juice.

Avocados: Choose avocados that are tender to the touch but not too soft. Too hard and they won't be ripe enough to eat.

Broccoli: Look for tight buds or florets; they indicate a fresher find.

Carrots and cucumbers: Think firm, not flabby.

Peppers (capsicums): Avoid peppers with wrinkled skin; it means they're starting to age.

Tomatoes: When possible, buy vine-ripened rather than hothouse. You don't have to be a gourmand to notice the improvement in taste and texture.

Bagged mixed salad leaves: The more colours, the more antioxidants. Look for one with red radicchio, pale green endive and dark green spinach.

Bagged baby spinach leaves: Peer through the bottom of the bag. If you see any mush, choose another one.

Spring onions, onions and garlic: Spring onions are much easier to use than whole onions for small meals – no half-cut-up, plastic-wrapped onions stinking up your fridge. For the same reason, buy small onions – which should be hard, not spongy when you squeeze them. Fresh garlic is firm and white or pinkish; avoid sad-looking yellowish bulbs, or bulbs with green shoots.

Fresh coriander: Tear off a leaf and taste it to make sure you're buying coriander and not flat-leaf parsley. Unless you don't like coriander. In that case, buy flat-leaf parsley and use it instead.

Nuts: Buy unroasted and unsalted loose nuts so you're not getting more sodium than you bargain for.

Meat: Your Muscle Maker

While turkey is a top-shelf Powerfood, that doesn't mean other meats are off-limits. The key is getting the leanest protein for the least amount of saturated fat. Turkey does the job exceptionally well, and chicken is almost as good. Breast meat is the lowest in fat, but the dark meat has twice as much iron and still only half the fat of lean beef.

Fresh turkey or chicken breasts: Check the label for sodium; some raw meats are plumped with a sodium solution – added salt you don't need. Look for one that contains less than 10 per cent water.

Minced turkey and chicken: If it's not made from breast meat, it could have as much fat as minced beef: check the label.

Precooked chicken: Check the label: the words 'chopped chicken' tell you it will have that strange chicken-from-concentrate texture. Avoid painted-on grill stripes.

Deli slices: For a little less sodium, choose plain or honey-roasted ham and turkey over smoked flavours.

Fresh salmon and other fish: Ask for wild-caught fish; it has fewer chemicals than farmed fish.

Smoked salmon: This is a high-sodium food, courtesy of the smoking. Pick the one with the lowest levels.

Steak: Pick the meat with the bluest tinge. That means it's aged enough for extra flavour, but it's not too old. Fillet and sirloin steak have the least fat.

Lean minced (ground) beef: You want 90 per cent lean (95 per cent lean if you can get it); it's the one with the least amount of saturated fat.

Back bacon: Buy lean back bacon rather than streaked-with-fat streaky, and go for thin-sliced rashers to help you keep the sodium tab down.

Pork loin cuts: Get the thin-cut ones; they cook in half the time.

Dairy: The Great White Help

Dairy products play a key role in the Abs Diet – as snacks, drinks, and as important ingredients in smoothies. They're your greatest

THE BEST PREPARED FOOD YOU CAN BUY. PERIOD.

Rotisserie chicken is an amazing thing. Not only does it look impressive, but it's an incredibly smart buy, both for the diet- and budget-conscious. First, always purchase a plain one; you're going to pick the skin off anyway, since that's where most of the fat hides. A breast and a leg will make a fine meal (check out the nutrition numbers below). Use the meat that's left to make a chicken salad or stuff it into a wrap. And then toss the entire carcass into a stockpot full of water with chopped vegetables and spices of your choice, simmer for a couple of hours, and you'll wind up with the best chicken soup you've ever eaten. (Just fish out the bones before digging in.)

90 g/3 oz breast meat (without skin)
138 calories/577 kJ, 3 g fat (2 g saturated), 65 mg sodium

90 g/3 oz dark meat (without skin)
176 calories/757 kJ, 9 g fat (2 g saturated), 80 mg sodium

source of calcium – the mineral more and more studies point to as a key weight-loss ingredient – and pack a potent protein punch as well. Think of the dairy section as fat-loss central. If you play the percentages.

Skimmed milk: Go organic. Cow antibiotics are for sick cows.

Chocolate milk: Choose cartons of low-fat long-life chocolate milk. They don't require refrigeration, so you can take a healthy source of calcium and protein with you anywhere.

Eggs: Omega-3 fortified eggs provide an extra shot of heart-healthy omega-3 fatty acids.

Low-fat and fat-free yogurt: Rachel's and Yeo Valley organic yogurts have the just-right creamy texture. In Australia, Jalna and Vaalia are good.

Ricotta cheese: Ricotta is a great natural source of whey protein, one of nature's premium muscle-builders. Buy a reduced-fat or light version if you can, but even the regular kind has only 11 per cent fat – or around 5 grams of fat per serving.

Cottage cheese and light soft cheese: These are stealth-sodium foods: choose brands with no added sodium and save the salt for something else.

Cheese sticks, slices and 'minis': Look for brands with the most protein and the least fat, but ones you like the taste of.

Smoothies: The Innocent and PJ brands contain no high-fructose corn syrup, which can't be said for all bottled smoothies.

Drinks: Liquid Assets

Loading up on fizzy drinks or fruit juice is like reverse liposuction; it's pouring calories that'll be stored as fat back into your body. There's only one drink of choice, but you can spruce it up with a slice of lemon or lime.

Bottled water: Buy an entire case. That way, you can't ignore it. Take a bottle everywhere.

Canned Foods: What's in Storage

Canned foods will outlast your grandchildren, which is why they're used for currency in so many postapocalypse movies. Just watch out for sodium, the main preservative.

Tuna: Go for tuna packed in water. Water cuts the fat.

Salmon: Choose wild red Pacific salmon rather than pink.

Chickpeas, black beans, kidney beans, lentils: You can't go wrong. But before you cook with them, always rinse off the salty solution they're soaked in.

Canned tomatoes: Make sure the brand you buy has no added salt/sodium, sugar or other sweeteners.

Sauces: Topping the List

Normally, sauces are like one-night stands. You enjoy them in the moment, but you feel pretty guilty afterwards. But I've uncovered some choice selections that might just make you interested in a lifelong commitment.

Olive oil: Choose extra virgin, which means the goods haven't been damaged by mixing with other oils.

Balsamic or red wine vinegar: There's no need to buy super-pricey vintage-dated vinegars, but it lasts for years, so you may as well get a decent drop.

Soy sauce: Amoy Reduced-Salt and Kikkoman Less Salt are two of the good guys: most varieties contain so much sodium it's like being buried in a salt mine.

Hot pepper sauce: Potent stuff: a drop or two of Tabasco should be plenty and the bottle will last forever.

Pasta sauces: There are some good, tomato-packed sauces out there – right next to the kind that are loaded with sugar, salt and chemicals. Choose sauces with around 5 g of fat or less per 100 g.

Mayonnaise: Hellmann's Extra Light Mayonnaise is one of the tastiest of the low-fat mayos, with just 6 per cent fat. Some brands are even lower in fat: they're labelled 97% fat-free.

Mustard: To me, Dijon-style mustards have a better flavour than the sharp yellow kinds, but you really can't go wrong.

Salsa: Most have only 2 g of fat per 100 g, so with that in mind, buy the one you like the taste of.

Peanut butter: The Whole Earth brand tastes exactly like roast peanuts. Not surprising, since peanuts – and a touch of salt (0.4 g per 100 g) – are its only ingredients. In Australia, the Sanitarium brand has no added salt, just a touch of oil.

Hummus: Some brands include roasted red peppers (capsicums), giving you a little extra flavour to go with the 3 grams of protein in a serving.

Chicken stock: Reduced-sodium or low-salt stock (fresh or canned) is worth looking out for. Joubère fresh stock tastes like the chicken, not like the container it came in. And it's low in sodium.

Bakery/Grains: The Incredible Bulk

Fibre is crucial to weight loss, and the best place to find it is in wholegrain baked goods. If the first ingredient isn't 'whole grain', 'wholemeal' or 'wholewheat', keep looking.

THE LOW-FAT BUZZWORDS

Remember, food labelling isn't about education, it's about marketing. Labels can be confusing, misleading and damaging if you don't know what you're getting into, especially when you're trying to figure out fat content. Here are some common phrases you'll see on food labels, and a look at what, exactly, they mean.

Regular: Greater than 3 grams of fat per 100 g

Reduced fat: 25 per cent less fat than the standard product

Light or lite: One-third fewer calories or 50 per cent less fat than normal

Low fat: No more than 3 grams of fat per 100 g

Non-fat or fat-free: Less than 0.15 gram of fat per 100 g

Wholemeal bread: Dove's Farm and Duchy Originals both offer a variety of high-fibre wholemeal breads. Australian brands include Tip Top and Buttercup Hyfibre.

Muffins: Wholemeal types have more fibre than white ones.

Pitta bread: Again, wholemeal types offer more fibre – about 3 grams per pitta – than white kinds.

Tortillas/wraps: Wholewheat tortillas are not available everywhere: if you can't find them, pick the tortilla with the most fibre and the least hydrogenated fat.

Pasta: De Cecco Whole Wheat is high in fibre, and this brand cooks well.

Brown rice: Uncle Ben's Wholegrain Rice is ready twice as fast as any other.

Cereal: Here's your best chance for fibre. My favourites include: Nature's Path Optimum Power Cereal (10 g of fibre per serving) and Kellogg's Bran Flakes (4.5 g).

Oats: If your need is speed, choose Quick Quaker Oats, Oatso Simple or Uncle Tobys Quick Oats. They cook in 1–3 minutes and deliver around 3 grams of fibre per serving. If you have a little more time, buy rolled oats. They take 7 to 9 minutes in the microwave, but they pack even more fibre per serving.

Baking: Piece of Cake

You'll have to navigate past the muffin mix and cake icing to find some important ingredients. Just grab your nuts and get outta there fast.

LOOK! DOWN THERE! IT'S A BARGAIN!

More expensive items are typically found at eye level – right where you'll see them and sweep them into the trolley without thinking. Look down, though, and you're likely to find a lower-priced version of the same thing.

Nuts: Choose flaked almonds, chopped pecans, crushed walnuts – anything that'll slip into a bowl of porridge or a smoothie and help save you time on the chopping block.

Honey: Buy the in-store brand. You'll use only small amounts, so there's no point in buying the super-expensive ones.

Spices: Here's another case where value rules. Despite what the label says, they'll last for ages, not just a couple of months. Get the cheap ones. You'll need dried basil, ground ginger, cinnamon, cumin and paprika.

Biscuits and Confectionery: No-Sweat Sweets

Spend too much time here and you'll get fatter just thinking about all the sugar, high-fructose corn syrup and trans fats that are lurking in these products. You'll have plenty of opportunity to satisfy sweet cravings – especially with smoothies that taste like shakes. But slip down this aisle for a few necessities.

Biscuits: Fig rolls – they're sweet and satisfying, thanks to the fibre: there's 1 gram of fibre in 2 fig rolls.

Chocolate: Pick up Snickers in the bite-sized bags. The key part is bite-sized. Or a box of After Eight mints – yes, they're wafer-thin. Enjoying one or two after dinner is a pleasure no one should be deprived of, diet or not. You just have to supply the willpower to keep it at one or two.

Crackers and crispbread: Ryvita Crispbreads, Misura Wholegrain crackers (from Italy) and Vita-Weat in Australia are the best wholewheat crackers for fibre.

Health Food: Alternative Routes

Most foods in the health food aisle or shop taste like the box your computer came in – only worse. (Rice cakes? No thanks.) But there are some great finds lurking in the aisles, and you don't have to be a dietary masochist or an unreformed hippie to shop for them.

Flaxseed: Buying your flax pre-ground saves time. And if you can find one that comes in a 455-g/1-lb container, it'll last for months. Look for it in the refrigerated section.

Whey protein: Look for protein powder that also includes casein, another dairy-based muscle builder.

Ready-Prepared Foods

Remember when you were a kid, and all you had to do to score a heaped plateful of shepherd's pie and green beans was show up at

LABELLING LESSON

Any food label is like a store window. The front of it is designed to draw you in, and then once you're inside, you can figure out whether the product is worth it. With a food label, once you get past the pretty colours and the coquettish cartoon mermaid, you need to flip the can over and inspect the label. Here's what to look for.

Serving size: How much you consume. A common trick is for something that appears to be one serving (a bottled drink) to actually be two or more. Don't be fooled.

Calories/kilojoules: The measure of energy a food provides. Calories mean different things depending on what you eat, but in the end, extra calories that your body can't burn will get stored as fat.

Fat: It's the combined total of saturated, polyunsaturated, monounsat urated and trans fats. Look for a ratio that's at least 3 to 1, total to sat urated. If monos and polys are listed, it's probably a healthy food. If it's more than 33 per cent saturated or trans fat, consider an alternative.

Sodium: A mineral (salt, basically) added for flavour and to preserve foods. Unless you have high blood pressure or are sodium sensitive, use 2,000 mg (2 g) as a reasonable daily target. More than that will not only raise your risk of hypertension (high blood pressure), it will also make you retain water and look and feel heavier.

Total carbohydrate: This includes all of the sugar and starch. Total number isn't as important as the kind.

the dinner table? The expanded deli sections of most supermarkets operate on the same principle. They cook it; you eat it. But this section of the supermarket is as littered with nutritional land mines as the rest (yeah, I mean you). Here's how to chart a healthy path.

Heat-and-Eat Meals

ABS DIET ENDORSEMENT:

Tuscan chicken (tomato and basil sauce) 205 calories/858 kJ, 6 g fat (2 g saturated), 2.5 g fibre

Fibre: The roughage that cleans your digestive and circulatory system. Insoluble fibre (in wholegrain foods, nuts and beans) expands and takes up space in your stomach, so it makes you feel full. Soluble fibre (in fruit, vegetables and oats) keeps blood vessels lubricated so cholesterol won't stick. Almost any food with at least 2 grams of fibre per serving is good. Five is even better.

Protein: Amino acids that build and maintain your entire body. It helps you feel satisfied. Men who exercise should aim for 162 to 225 grams per day – and women around 100. Thinner men need no more than 114 grams. Thinner women around 75.

Vitamin and mineral percentages: The food's percentage of the minimum amounts of nutrients required to prevent various deficiency diseases. As long as you're eating the ABS DIET POWER 12, you should be getting all the vitamins and minerals you need, but it never hurts to take a daily multivitamin for extra insurance.

Ingredients: Arranged in order by weight from most to least. Bad foods like high-fructose corn syrup, glucose syrup and partially hydrogenated oils should be the fifth ingredient listed or lower. If not, move on.

Cholesterol: It's a fatlike substance from animal products, and it's found in all our cell membranes. Your body manufactures most of your cholesterol; what food adds is only a small percentage. Don't worry about it and don't get drawn in by otherwise unhealthy foods that claim 'no cholesterol'. As a nutritional selling point, it's worthless.

THE LESSER OF TWO EVILS

Eat this: *Salmon fishcakes* 296 calories/1240 kJ, 16 g fat (3 g saturated), 1.5 g fibre

Not that: *Fish in breadcrumbs* 360 calories/1507 kJ, 20 g fat (3 g saturated), 1.5 g fibre

Eat this: *Chilli con carne with rice* 400 calories/1674 kJ, 15 g fat (5 g saturated), 2.5 g fibre

Not that: *Lasagne* 600 calories/2512 kJ, 25 g fat (11 g saturated), 1.5 g fibre

Heat-and-Eat Vegetables

ABS DIET ENDORSEMENTS:

Ratatouille 82 calories/343 kJ, 3.5 g fat (1 g saturated), 1 g fibre

Stuffed pepper (capsicum) 175 calories/732 kJ, 5 g fat (3 g saturated), 1.2 g fibre

THE LESSER OF TWO EVILS

Eat this: *Cauliflower cheese* 200 calories/837 kJ, 12.5 g fat (6 g saturated), 2.5 g fibre

Not that: *Potato gratin* 360 calories/1506 kJ, 25 g fat (12 g saturated), 1.5 g fibre

Salads

ABS DIET ENDORSEMENTS:

Mixed bean salad 150 calories/628 kJ, 6 g fat (0 g saturated), 5 g fibre

Caesar salad 185 calories/775 kJ, 13 g fat (4 g saturated), 1 g fibre

THE LESSER OF TWO EVILS

Eat this: *Pasta salad with vegetables* 200 calories/837 kJ, 15 g fat (5 g saturated), 2.5 g fibre

Not that: *Potato salad* 300 calories/1256 kJ, 26 g fat (15 g saturated), 1.5 g fibre

FAT CONTENT OF MEAT (115 G/4 OZ, RAW, WITHOUT SKIN OR BONE)

	TOTAL FAT (G)	SATURATED (G)
Turkey breast	1	0.3
Skinless chicken breast	1.2	0.4
Venison	1.8	0.7
Veal steak or escalope	1.9	0.7
Wild rabbit	2.6	0.8
Turkey leg	2.8	0.9
Chicken drumstick	3.2	0.9
Cured ham	4.7	1.5
Lean beef rump steak	4.7	2
Lean beef sirloin steak	5.1	2
Lean pork tenderloin/fillet	5.7	1.6
Lean ham/gammon	6	2
Lean minced turkey	6.9	2.9
Beef fillet steak	7	3
Duck breast	7.4	2.3
Lean pork chop	8.2	2.8
Lean lamb (loin, leg)	9.5	4
Lean minced beef	11	4.6
Rib-eye steak	18	7.3
Beef fore-rib/rib roast	19.8	10.2
Pork belly	60.1	21.9

The Freezer: Cold Comfort

Make this your last stop when shopping and you'll likely make it home with your ice cream intact. 'Ice cream?' you say. Right. This plan is designed for human beings rather than robots.

Prawns: Since prawns can be expensive, just pick the least expensive. There's no real difference.

Berries and fruit: If you're buying frozen, it pays to go organic. Because they're delicate, berries and fruit often top the lists of high-pesticide produce.

Peas, spinach, sweetcorn: These often contain more vitamins than the fresh versions, so keep a stash in your freezer.

ABS DIET SUCCESS STORY

'IT DOESN'T EVEN FEEL LIKE A DIET'

Name: Jon Armond

Height: 1.94 m/6'4"

Age: 33

Weight, Week 1: 116 kg/18 st 2 lb

Weight, Week 6: 104 kg/16 st 5 lb

Weight, Week 9: 100 kg/15 st 9 lb

Body-Fat Percentage, Week 1: 27

Body-Fat Percentage, Week 9: 18

Jon Armond's a big guy, and he's always carried his weight well. When he told people he was trying to lose weight, they told him he didn't need to. But Armond knew better. Carrying more than 115 kg/18 st around everywhere he went was taking a serious toll on his body, and he knew he needed to drop some serious weight.

Even though he was active, Armond was one of those guys who rationalized that he could eat whatever he wanted because he had exercised.

Edamame (green soya beans): Make things easy for yourself and buy the already shelled kind.

Ice cream: Traditional ice creams have between 15 and 20 g of fat (mostly saturated) per 100 g, but there's a growing number of light ice creams with around one-third of the fat – some of them surprisingly luxurious.

Frozen Dinners

Frozen dinners can fit into nearly any diet for one reason: they're perfectly portion-controlled. In a study at the University of Illinois, people who regularly ate dinners from the freezer section

---

But the fact was that he ate and drank too much, and he was always tired. (He frequently took naps in the middle of the day.)

'I just didn't feel like I was 33,' he says. 'I felt like I was 53.' Then he found the Abs Diet.

'When I looked in *Men's Health* and looked at the way the Abs Diet was set up, something clicked. This made perfect sense,' he says. 'I knew I'd lose weight, but what I didn't expect was the total-body transformation – to see the fat drop and the muscle gain at the same time. That's what I really appreciate about it.'

For the first 6 weeks, Armond stuck to the principles without wavering, and he realized that it wasn't really a diet at all, but just a different approach to eating.

'I found myself not even consumed with it. I've never been on a diet that you didn't have to think about being on the diet all the time,' he says. Instead, it was a plan that he simply incorporated into his life, and by doing so, he's traded in his 'huge beer gut'.

'I've got some abs showing through now,' Armond says. 'I was wearing size 38s, and I just bought 34s. I was wearing extra, extra large shirts and now I'm wearing larges. I'm ready to go on the public-speaking circuit to talk about the Abs Diet.'

lost 31 per cent more weight than their free-eating counterparts. Like their counterparts in the chilled meals section, many frozen meals these days are aimed specifically at people interested in weight loss. Whichever brand you choose, aim for a maximum of 10 to 15 g of fat per serving – make sure you're not reading the fat content per 100g – and pay attention to the amount of saturated fat. You also need to check that they're not too high in sodium – a hidden danger of the freezer aisle. Happily, some manufacturers are becoming more aware of the importance of fibre. Supermarket own-brands change their recipes frequently, and are increasingly imaginative in the meals they offer.

Weight Watchers

A world leader in this category, with dozens of virtually fat-free meals. Widely available, the range varies from shop to shop.

Birds Eye Steam Fresh (UK only)

ABS DIET SUCCESS STORY

A FORMER ATHLETE FINDS A BETTER BODY

Name: Mark Peterson

Age: 25

Height: 1.75 m/5'9"

Weight, Week 1: 85 kg/13 st 5 lb

Weight, Week 6: 77 kg/12 st 2 lb

Weight, Week 12: 74 kg/11 st 10 lb

Mark Peterson was a swimmer in school and competed in triathlons. But then all that eating during college and law school hit him.

'Law school is the most unhealthy thing I've ever done in my life,' he says. 'I was looking for something to get me back in shape.'

Lean Cuisine
Lean Beef Lasagne
Chicken Cacciatore
Thai Style Chicken Curry with Rice

SlimFast (UK only)
Beef Casserole with Rice
Chicken Korma with Coriander and Basmati Rice
Thai Chicken with Lemongrass and Rice

UK supermarket own-brand ranges:
Asda Good for you!
Iceland Good Choice
Marks & Spencer Count On Us
Sainsbury's Be Good To Yourself
Tesco Healthy Living
Waitrose Perfectly Balanced

He decided to train for the Chicago marathon and found a diet to support his training.

'The Abs Diet gave you a lot of different foods that you could have,' he says. 'It just seemed like a diet you could totally stick to.'

He lived on almonds as a snack, spinach salad as lunch, peanut butter on wholemeal toast before his workout, and made chicken or fish for dinner. 'I didn't like porridge, so I substituted Kashi and Go Lean cereals.'

In the autumn, Peterson completed the marathon, and friends who hadn't seen him for months noticed the transformation. 'They all said that it looked like I didn't need to lose weight, but it's totally different when they see me now. A lot of friends couldn't believe the weight I lost.'

Now that marathon training is over, he has another goal in mind. 'I swam like crazy in school, and I focused a lot on running, but I've never been close to a six-pack,' he says. 'This is the closest I've ever been.'

Chapter 5

LET'S GET IT STARTED

24 Abs Diet Breakfasts

BEFORE WORK, there's a lot to do – take a shower, check the weather, dress the kids, glance at the stocks and shares, brush your teeth, zip your trousers. In that routine, there's not much you can sacrifice – unless you want go to work in your underpants. So many of us end up treating breakfast like it's a luxury – something that we do only if we have time or if there's a slice of bread near the toaster. But sacrificing breakfast is like arguing with the cops; there's absolutely nothing good that can come of it. Without breakfast, you're operating on reserves, putting your body in a pseudostarvation mode that tells your body's metabolism to slow down to protect you. What you need to do is eat – and eat heartily. Since I know you've apportioned about as much time to make breakfast as you have to slide on your socks, I've whipped up some recipes you can zip through faster than those artery-clogged lines at the drive-through.

So fire 'em up and start the day strong. What you eat the first hour you're awake will have a huge effect on what you eat for the next 16 or 17. I'm a firm believer that if every day of good eating is a race, then how well you start determines how well you finish.

Quicker Oats

USE PLAIN INSTANT OATS for the following recipes. Nothing personal, Quaker guy, but those powdery sugared packets are as antiquated as that hat. For each recipe, mix all ingredients in a microwave-safe bowl and nuke for 2 minutes, unless otherwise noted. All serve 1.

Honey, I Shrunk My Gut (Powerfoods: 4)

240 ml/8 fl oz skimmed milk

60 g/2 oz plain instant oats

75 g/2½ oz blue- or blackberries

1 tablespoon chopped walnuts or pecans

1 teaspoon honey

1 teaspoon ground flaxseed

Pinch of ground cinnamon

Per serving: 472 cals/1985 kJ, 19 g protein, 62 g carbohydrates, 18 g fat (2 g saturated), 7 g fibre, 140 mg sodium

Flax Machine (Powerfoods: 4)

240 ml/8 fl oz skimmed milk

60 g/2 oz plain instant oats

½ banana, sliced

1 tablespoon peanut butter

1 teaspoon honey

1 teaspoon ground flaxseed

Pinch of brown sugar

Per serving: 487 cals/2052 kJ, 20 g protein, 71 g carbohydrates, 16 g fat (3 g saturated), 5.5 g fibre, 190 mg sodium

You're Nuts (Powerfoods: 5)

240 ml/8 fl oz skimmed milk

60 g/2 oz plain instant oats

1 tablespoon chopped pecans

1 tablespoon chopped walnuts

1½ teaspoons honey

1 teaspoon ground flaxseed

⅛ teaspoon ground cinnamon

Per serving: 568 cals/2382 kJ, 19 g protein, 62 g carbohydrates, 29 g fat (3 g saturated), 5.5 g fibre, 139 mg sodium

Ginger? Roger! (Powerfoods: 5)

240 ml/8 fl oz skimmed milk

60 g/2 oz plain instant oats

1 tablespoon sliced almonds

1 teaspoon honey

1 teaspoon ground flaxseed

½ teaspoon ground ginger

1 tablespoon vanilla yogurt

Mix milk, oats, almonds, honey, flaxseed and ginger in a microwave-safe bowl. Nuke for 2 minutes. Top with yogurt.

Per serving: 475 cals/2006 kJ, 20 g protein, 64 g carbohydrates, 17 g fat (2 g saturated), 5.5 g fibre, 141 mg sodium

Instant Omelettes

At a café, an omelette is just code for 'throw the leftovers in a pan with some eggs'. At home, they're a quick source of protein – and a chance to boost your Powerfood count with one pan only. For all recipes, stir 2 eggs with a fork until white and yolk are well blended. Add the remaining ingredients. Nuke for 2 minutes and 30 seconds or until the eggs are firmly set. All serve 1.

Tom Tomelette (Powerfoods: 3)

> 2 eggs
> 1 (15 g/½ oz) slice turkey, diced
> 1 tablespoon grated reduced-fat Cheddar cheese

Per serving: 213 cals/888 kJ, 22 g protein, 0 g carbohydrates, 14 g fat (5 g saturated), 0 g fibre, 248 mg sodium

The Green and White (Powerfoods: 3)

> 2 eggs
> 1 tablespoon grated reduced-fat mozzarella cheese

15 g/½ oz baby spinach leaves, torn

Per serving: 193 cals/803 kJ, 16 g protein, 0.2 g carbohydrates, 14 g fat (5 g saturated), 0.3 g fibre, 220 mg sodium

Lean Eggs and Ham (Powerfoods: 2)

> 2 eggs
> 1 rasher back bacon, grilled, then diced
> 1 slice tomato, chopped

Per serving: 225 cals/936 kJ, 18 g protein, 0.5 g carbohydrates, 16 g fat (5 g saturated), 0.1 g fibre, 611 mg sodium

Bean Counter (Powerfoods: 2)

> 2 eggs
> 2 tablespoons rinsed canned black beans
> 1 teaspoon chopped fresh coriander

After cooking, top with 1 tablespoon salsa.

Per serving: 197 cals/825 kJ, 16 g protein, 8 g carbohydrates, 11 g fat (3 g saturated), 1.5 g fibre, 142 mg sodium

Up in Smoke (Powerfoods: 3)

2 eggs

30 g/1 oz smoked salmon, chopped

15 g/½ oz baby spinach leaves, torn

Per serving: 197 cals/822 kJ, 20 g protein, 0.2 g carbohydrates, 12.5 g fat (3.5 g saturated), 0.3 g fibre, 725 mg sodium

Mister Bean (Powerfoods: 4)

2 eggs

1 (15 g/½ oz) slice turkey, diced

1 tablespoon rinsed canned black or cannellini beans

1 tablespoon grated reduced-fat mozzarella cheese

Per serving: 236 cals/983 kJ, 22 g protein, 4 g carbohydrates, 15 g fat (5.5 g saturated), 0.5 g fibre, 208 mg sodium

Breakfast Tortillas

You usually eat tortillas or wraps for lunch, but a tortilla is one of the easiest things you can make for breakfast. Just arrange all the ingredients on the tortilla, fold the ends, then neatly roll. For recipes that call for nuked eggs, you can scramble them in about 60 seconds. In a microwave-safe bowl, stir the eggs with a fork until white and yolk are well blended and then bung them into the microwave.

Holy Guacamole! (Powerfoods: 5)

1 medium wholewheat tortilla

2 (15 g/½ oz each) slices turkey

2 nuked eggs

½ avocado, sliced

2 tablespoon grated reduced-fat Cheddar cheese

Per serving: 481 cals/2014 kJ, 37 g protein, 25 g carbohydrates, 26 g fat (8 g saturated), 1.5 g fibre, 425 mg sodium

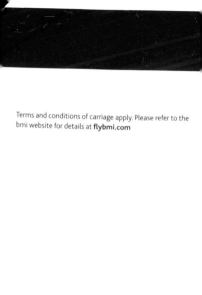

Terms and conditions of carriage apply. Please refer to the bmi website for details at **flybmi.com**

bmi boarding pass

name of passenger

CRAIK/LINDA

ETKT 0862124211003

from **LHR**

to **SFO**

VIRGIN ATLANTIC

carrier   flight no. / class   date

VS 019   X 27SEP

gate	gate closes	seat
. . . .	0945	48A

pcs.   ck. wt.   unck. wt. pcs.   ck. wt.   unck. wt.

Yosemite Salmon (Powerfoods: 6)

2 tablespoons low-fat soft cheese or ricotta cheese

1 medium wholewheat tortilla

30 g/1 oz smoked salmon, torn into little pieces

2 nuked eggs

30 g/1 oz baby spinach, chopped

1 spring onion, sliced

Spread the cheese on the tortilla, then arrange the remaining ingredients, fold the ends in, and roll.

Per serving: 367 cals/1540 kJ, 31 g protein, 26 g carbohydrates, 16 g fat (6 g saturated), 0.5 g fibre, 988 mg sodium

Huevos Rancheros (Powerfoods: 4)

1 medium wholewheat tortilla

2 nuked eggs

1 spring onion, sliced

1 tablespoon chopped fresh coriander

2 tablespoons grated reduced-fat Cheddar cheese

2 tablespoons salsa

Per serving: 359 cals/1505 kJ, 26.5 g protein, 28 g carbohydrates, 16 g fat (6 g saturated), 0.5 g fibre, 408 mg sodium

DAIRY DAIRY, QUITE CONTRARY

At breakfast, put coffee in your milk instead of milk in your coffee. Fill your mug to the rim with skimmed milk first thing in the morning. Drink it down until all that's left is the amount you'd normally add to your coffee; then pour your java on top. You just took in 25 per cent of the vitamin D you need every day and 30 per cent of the calcium.

Breakfast Sandwiches

Once suitable only for the lunch box, today sandwiches might show up anywhere – as fancy canapés, as hearty dinners, as sexual fantasies . . . OK, let's not go there. Right now we're concentrating on breakfast, so let's take a look at some healthy choices you can serve up in the morning. (Who you serve them to is your business.)

Eggs-cellent Adventure (Powerfoods: 3)

> 1 tablespoon salsa
>
> 1 toasted wholemeal muffin
>
> 1 nuked egg
>
> 1 teaspoon chopped fresh coriander
>
> 1 tablespoon grated reduced-fat Cheddar cheese

ABS DIET SUCCESS STORY

HE LOST WEIGHT AND CURED HIS PAIN

Name: John Kelly

Age: 40

Height: 1.85 m/6'1"

Weight, Week 1: 98 kg/15 st 5 lb

Weight, Week 6: 88 kg/13 st 11 lb

When John Kelly was diagnosed with Barrett's disease – a condition caused by chronic acid reflux that can lead to oesophageal cancer – he knew something had to change. He had a demanding job, three sons under the age of 9, and the stress of moving to a new house.

'It's hard to take care of yourself when there are so many other responsibilities that dominate your life,' he says. Caught up in trying to be all things to all people, Kelly let his diet and exercise programme slide, and, no surprise, he gained weight. 'I just thought that gaining weight and being tired were par for the course.'

Spread salsa on one half of the muffin, top with the egg, coriander and cheese. Toast under the grill until the cheese melts.

Per serving: 311 cals/1309 kJ, 19 g protein, 38 g carbohydrates, 10 g fat (3 g saturated), 1.5 g fibre, 525 mg sodium

Foxy Lox (Powerfoods: 3)

    2 tablespoons low-fat soft cheese or ricotta cheese
    1 toasted wholemeal muffin
    1 slice tomato
  30 g/1 oz smoked salmon

Spread cheese over each muffin half, top with tomato and salmon.

Per serving: 286 cals/1208 kJ, 22 g protein, 38 g carbohydrates, 6.5 g fat (2.5 g saturated), 1.5 g fibre, 1096 mg sodium

But what wasn't par for the course were the unexplained pains in his chest. The pain was building to the point where he'd feel nauseous three times a week, and it got so bad that he had to skip work sometimes. When his doctor diagnosed Barrett's disease, Kelly began searching for ways to change his lifestyle, and he found some in the Abs Diet.

Because of the limitations he had with his illness – no fatty meats, spicy foods or tomato sauce – Kelly found that the Abs Diet worked for him.

'My condition meant no vices – no alcohol or caffeine – so the idea of a diet that featured daily smoothies was pretty appealing,' Kelly says.

Within weeks, the fat began to melt, and the muscles appeared. But it wasn't just the fat – or the fact that his energy levels had increased. Kelly hasn't experienced any symptoms since starting the diet.

'The Abs Diet helped me return to a more normal life on so many levels that the weight loss and fitness gain are just the icing on the cake,' Kelly says. 'Being able to contribute at my job and participate in my boys' lives more actively are blessings that I could have never imagined could come from a diet.'

The Big Breakfast (Powerfoods: 4)

- 1 nuked egg
- 1 rasher back bacon, grilled
- 1 slice tomato
- 1 toasted wholemeal muffin
- 1 tablespoon grated reduced-fat Cheddar cheese

Arrange the egg, bacon and tomato on one half of the muffin. Top with the cheese. Toast under the grill until the cheese melts.
Per serving: 377 cals/1584 kJ, 25 g protein, 37 g carbohydrates, 15 g fat (5 g saturated), 1.5 g fibre, 997 mg sodium

Apple Jacked (Powerfoods: 4)

- 1 toasted wholemeal muffin
- 1 rasher back bacon, grilled
- 2 slices apple
- 2 tablespoons peanut butter

Per serving: 456 cals/1909 kJ, 21 g protein, 44 g carbohydrates, 23 g fat (6 g saturated), 3.5 g fibre, 931 mg sodium

Jam Session (Powerfoods: 3)

- 1 toasted wholemeal muffin
- 2 tablespoons low-fat soft cheese or ricotta cheese
- 50 g/1¾ oz blue-, black- or raspberries, slightly crushed (mash berries in small bowl with fork)

Per serving: 253 cals/1072 kJ, 15 g protein, 40 g carbohydrates, 5 g fat (2.5 g saturated), 2.5 g fibre, 532 mg sodium

Power PB (Powerfoods: 3)

- 1 slice wholemeal bread
- 2 tablespoons peanut butter
- 40 g/1¼ oz blue-, black- or raspberries, slightly crushed

Toast the bread. Spread the peanut butter on the toast and cut in half. Add the berries to one half, then cover with the other half and squeeze lightly.

Per serving: 257 cals/1073 kJ, 10 g protein, 18 g carbohydrates, 16.5 g fat (4 g saturated), 4 g fibre, 252 mg sodium

Turk before Work (Powerfoods: 3)

1 slice wholemeal bread

2 (15 g/½ oz each) slices turkey

2 slices apple

Toast the bread. Arrange the turkey and apple on the toast, then fold lightly in half.

Per serving: 125 cals/531 kJ, 13 g protein, 16 g carbohydrates, 1.5 g fat (0.3 g saturated), 2 g fibre, 162 mg sodium

Turbocharged Yogurt

In case you missed it (and I don't know how, since I've been jumping up and down and waving my arms about it for nearly 100 pages now), calcium is one of those ingredients that fortifies more than your skeleton. It seems to be a potent player in the weight-loss game. At breakfast, yogurt is the fastest power player since Andy Roddick. For all, just mix the ingredients and eat.

Bananarama (Powerfoods: 2)

225 g/8 oz vanilla yogurt

1 banana, sliced

1 tablespoon chopped walnuts

Per serving: 382 cals/1612 kJ, 12 g protein, 59 g carbohydrates, 12.5 g fat (2 g saturated), 1.5 g fibre, 148 mg sodium

Berry Easy (Powerfoods: 3)

225 g/8 oz low-fat natural yogurt

75 g/2½ oz mixed berries

1 teaspoon ground flaxseed

Per serving: 167 cals/707 kJ, 13.5 g protein, 20 g carbohydrates, 4.5 g fat (1 g saturated), 2 g fibre, 190 mg sodium

A Trip to the Peach (Powerfoods: 2)

225 g/8 oz vanilla yogurt

75 g/2½ oz frozen or canned in juice, drained, peaches

1 tablespoon flaked almonds

Per serving: 324 cals/1368 kJ, 12 g protein, 49 g carbohydrates, 10 g fat (2 g saturated), 1.5 g fibre, 157 mg sodium

The Super Bowl of Breakfasts

Eight power foods in one bowl? We haven't seen this many A-listers since Oscar night. Start mixing.

The Ultimate Power Breakfast (Powerfoods: 8)

1 egg

240 ml/8 fl oz skimmed milk

60 g/2 oz instant oats

75 g/2½ oz mixed berries

1 tablespoon chopped pecans or flaked almonds

1 teaspoon vanilla whey protein powder

1 teaspoon ground flaxseed

½ banana, sliced

1 tablespoon low-fat natural yogurt

In a microwave-safe bowl, mix the egg well, then add the next 6 ingredients and nuke for 2 minutes. Remove from the microwave and allow to cool for a minute or two. Top with the sliced banana and yogurt.

Per serving: 592 cals/2491 kJ, 27 g protein, 69 g carbohydrates, 25 g fat (4 g saturated), 7.5 g fibre, 218 mg sodium

Chapter 6

LEAN IN THE MIDDLE

25 Abs Diet Lunches

DEPENDING ON WHAT you do during the day, lunch can often present you with the opportunity to blow your diet like a tropical storm through the Florida Keys. Lunch comes at the very time of day when forces outside our control are vying for our time. If your job is demanding, lunch sometimes means you have 3 minutes to pop a snack out of the machine and get back to your desk. If you work with the get-some-fresh-air types, you're on the road at 12 and ordering a burger and beer by 12:06. If you need to have fancy business lunches, you're susceptible to the onslaught of free bread, creamy sauces and four-storey desserts. If you're home with the kids, you're one temper tantrum away from a macaroni cheese binge.

That's why I suggest that if there's one meal that you should plan every day, it's lunch. Preparing for it makes you less likely to fall victim to any one of the diet busters waiting to pounce. It doesn't matter whether you make your lunch the night before, in the morning or 3 minutes before you're going to eat it. The point is: preparation breeds motivation.

Wraps

The trend towards sandwich wraps over the past few years has made eating a healthy lunch easier than ever before. An easy-access tortilla cuts down on empty calories and eliminates the need for utensils. But there are some bum wraps out there, so I've rolled up and rolled out a handful of smart choices just packed with Powerfoods. All make 1 serving.

Thai One On (Powerfoods: 4)

1½ tablespoons peanut butter

1 wholewheat tortilla

100 g/3½ oz cooked chicken, chopped

45 g/1½ oz mixed salad leaves

30 g/1 oz carrots, cut into matchsticks

1 teaspoon chopped fresh coriander

Spread peanut butter down the centre of the tortilla. Add chicken and remaining ingredients. Fold outside edges in, then roll.

Per serving: 456 cals/1913 kJ, 39 g protein, 30 g carbohydrates, 20 g fat (5.5 g saturated), 214 g fibre, 241 mg sodium

Christmas Cracker (Powerfoods: 4)

2 tablespoons cranberry sauce

1 wholewheat tortilla

3 (15 g/½ oz each) slices turkey

30 g/1 oz Brie cheese

45 g/1½ oz mixed salad leaves

Spread cranberry sauce down the centre of the tortilla. Add turkey and remaining ingredients. Fold outside edges in, then roll.

Per serving: 346 cals/1461 kJ, 26 g protein, 40 g carbohydrates, 10 g fat (6 g saturated), 0.5 g fibre, 306 mg sodium

The Cow Tipper (Powerfoods: 3)

3 (15 g/½ oz each) slices roast beef

1 wholewheat tortilla

45 g/1½ oz mixed salad leaves

1– 2 tomatoes, chopped

1 tablespoon Dijon mustard

1 tablespoon crumbled blue cheese

Arrange beef slices down the centre of the tortilla, then add remaining ingredients. Fold outside edges in, then roll.

Per serving: 350 cals/1468 kJ, 20.5 g protein, 30 g carbohydrates, 17 g fat (8 g saturated), 1.5 g fibre, 664 mg sodium

The Two Turks (Powerfoods: 6)

2 (15 g/½ oz each) slices turkey

1 wholewheat tortilla

2 slices turkey bacon, cooked

45 g/1½ oz mixed salad leaves

3 slices avocado

2 tablespoons grated reduced-fat Cheddar cheese

Arrange turkey slices down the centre of the tortilla, then add remaining ingredients. Fold outside edges in, then roll.

Per serving: 348 cals/1465 kJ, 30 g protein, 27 g carbohydrates, 14 g fat (5 g saturated), 1.5 g fibre, 492 mg sodium

Hot Curlers (Powerfoods: 4)

1 tablespoon Dijon mustard

1 wholewheat tortilla

100 g/3½ oz cooked chicken, chopped

45 g/1½ oz mixed salad leaves

1–2 tomatoes, diced

Tabasco sauce, to taste

2 tablespoons grated reduced-fat Cheddar cheese

Spread the mustard down the centre of the tortilla. Add chicken and remaining ingredients. Fold outside edges in, then roll.

Per serving: 422 cals/1776 kJ, 45 g protein, 30 g carbohydrates, 14 g fat (5.5 g saturated), 1.5 g fibre, 805 mg sodium

Salads

Your standard chain-restaurant salad bar is a nutritional minefield – there are plenty of healthy, safe moves to make and plenty of fat bombs that can blow up your gut: potato salad, pasta salad, croutons, those bacon bits that look like gravel. If you make your own salad, you can ensure that your salad has taste and power. All make 1 serving.

The Olympiad (Powerfoods: 4)

150 g/5½ oz	mixed salad leaves
1	plum tomato, chopped
40 g/1¼ oz	cucumber, chopped
1	tablespoon grated reduced-fat mozzarella cheese
	Pinch of black pepper
1	tablespoon balsamic or red wine vinegar
1	teaspoon olive oil

Per serving: 180 cals/747 kJ, 5 g protein, 6 g carbohydrates, 15 g fat (4 g saturated), 2.5 g fibre, 74 mg sodium

DIY DRESSINGS

Ever wondered how something that should by all laws of nature be refrigerated – like blue cheese dressing – manages to stay out on shelves? Trans fat and lots of preservatives do the work, making salad dressings some of the biggest belly-bloating foods out there.

Making your own salad dressing is just a little bit harder than boiling water, but it will ensure that you're eating 100 per cent healthy (and it'll taste better, too). Add 1 part olive oil to 2 parts acid, such as lemon juice, orange juice, vinegar or wine. Stir together to blend or pour each one on the salad.

Sweet Cheeses! (Powerfoods: 5)

150 g/5½ oz mixed salad leaves

  75 g/2½ oz berries (any type or a mix)

          1 tablespoon chopped onion

          1 tablespoon crumbled blue cheese

          1 tablespoon chopped pecans or walnuts

          1 teaspoon ground flaxseed

          1 tablespoon balsamic vinegar

          1 teaspoon olive oil

Per serving: 281 cals/1168 kJ, 8 g protein, 8 g carbohydrates, 24 g fat (5.5 g saturated), 3.5 g fibre, 128 mg sodium

Orient Express (Powerfoods: 6)

150 g/5½ oz mixed salad leaves

  75 g/2½ oz cooked chicken, diced

          1 spring onion, sliced

          ½ green pepper (capsicum), chopped

          1 tablespoon flaked almonds

          1 teaspoon chopped fresh coriander

          1 tablespoon orange juice

          1 teaspoon olive oil

Per serving: 361 cals/1503 kJ, 27 g protein, 6 g carbohydrates, 26 g fat (4 g saturated), 3 g fibre, 72 mg sodium

Kidney Punch (Powerfoods: 3)

150 g/5½ oz mixed salad leaves

  75 g/2½ oz drained canned kidney beans

          1 tablespoon chopped onion

          1 tablespoon crumbled blue cheese

            Pinch of black pepper

          1 tablespoon red wine

          1 teaspoon olive oil

Per serving: 274 cals/1140 kJ, 10 g protein, 17.5 g carbohydrates,
17 g fat (5 g saturated), 6.5 g fibre, 417 mg sodium

Potion of the Ocean (Powerfoods: 6)

150 g/5½ oz mixed salad leaves

6 large prawns, cooked

1 spring onion, sliced

40 g/1¼ oz cucumber, chopped

½ green pepper (capsicum), chopped

1 tablespoon lemon juice

1 teaspoon olive oil

Per serving: 193 cals/803 kJ, 16 g protein, 5 g carbohydrates,
12.5 g fat (2 g saturated), 2 g fibre, 962 mg sodium

El Tequila Ensalada (Powerfoods: 5)

150 g/5½ oz mixed salad leaves

75 g/2½ oz drained canned black beans

1 plum tomato, chopped

1 spring onion, sliced

½ avocado, sliced

1 teaspoon chopped fresh coriander

1 tablespoon tequila or, for the less stout of heart, lime juice

1 teaspoon olive oil

Per serving: 332 cals/1387 kJ, 9 g protein, 25 g carbohydrates,
22 g fat (4 g saturated), 6.5 g fibre, 19 mg sodium

WEEKLY GRIND

Several of these recipes call for lemon juice. If you have real lemons to hand, you can use the rind for zest. Zest adds flavour and, according to a University of Arizona study, a tablespoon of it each week can help cut the risk of developing skin cancer by 30 per cent. Another handy tip: after using half a lemon for juice or zest, toss the rest down the drain and let it clean out your rank garbage disposal.

Sandwiches

As far as ease goes, nothing beats a sandwich. Bread, meat, eat. Still, as drive-throughs prove, just because something's easy doesn't mean it's smart. There are plenty of sandwich ingredients, from mile-high corned beef to do-nothing-for-you white bread, that simply don't stack up. Still, we love the sandwich. The trick is to incorporate as many Abs Diet Powerfoods into your concoctions as you can. That means some wholegrain bread, some lean meat and some leafy greens if you like. You want to build the ultimate power sandwich that's filling and more well rounded than Anna Nicole Smith (circa 2003). To shake things up, try making these substitutions without the extra layer of guilt.

SANDWICH	SUBSTITUTE THIS	FOR THAT	ABS DIET ADVANTAGE
Abs Diet BLT	Turkey bacon	Regular bacon	59 fewer calories
	Reduced-fat soured cream	Mayo	2 more grams protein
	Baby spinach	Iceberg lettuce	2 grams more fibre
	Wholegrain bread	White bread	
Abs Diet meatball sub	Turkey meatballs	Beef meatballs	194 fewer calories
	Reduced-fat mozzarella	Full-fat mozzarella	4 grams less saturated fat
	Wholemeal roll	White roll	1 gram more fibre
Abs Diet po boy	Defrosted frozen cooked prawns	Deep-fried prawns	379 fewer calories
	Reduced-fat soured cream	Rémoulade	3.5 grams less saturated fat
	Baby spinach	Iceberg lettuce	2 grams more fibre
	Wholemeal roll	White roll	
Abs Diet kebab	Lean roast beef	Lamb	14 fewer calories
	Reduced-fat yogurt	Full-fat yogurt	1.5 grams less saturated fat
	Wholemeal pitta	White pitta	1 gram more fibre

SANDWICH	SUBSTITUTE THIS	FOR THAT	ABS DIET ADVANTAGE
Abs Diet PB&J	Natural peanut butter	Trans-fatty kind	74 fewer calories
	Slightly crushed fresh berries	Sugary jam	1 gram less saturated fat
	Wholemeal bread	White bread	2 grams more fibre

Fill-in-the-Blank-Salad Sandwich (Powerfoods: 4)

170 g/6 oz salmon or tuna or 100 g/3½ oz cooked chicken, chopped

1 spring onion, sliced

45 g/1½ oz cucumber, finely diced

1 tablespoon reduced-fat soured cream or natural yogurt

2 teaspoons Dijon mustard

1 teaspoon lemon juice

⅛ teaspoon lemon zest

Salt and pepper, to taste

Mix everything together in a big bowl, stirring well to blend in the lemon juice and soured cream. Eat with salad leaves or wholewheat crackers.

Salmon: Per serving: 302 cals/1264 kJ, 37 g protein, 4 g carbohydrates, 15 g fat (2.5 g saturated), 0.5 g fibre, 1456 mg sodium

Tuna: Per serving: 207 cals/878 kJ, 42 g protein, 4 g carbohydrates, 2.5 g fat (0.5 g saturated), 0.5 g fibre, 1031 mg sodium

Chicken: Per serving: 221 cals/927 kJ, 32 g protein, 4 g carbohydrates, 9 g fat (2.5 g saturated), 0.5 g fibre, 569 mg sodium

Soups

Soup is not the kind of food you think of as fitting into a busy lifestyle, it's hard to stash in your briefcase, tough to eat on the train, and generally frowned upon at business meetings. But soup does offer one big convenience. You can whip up a batch, store it in the fridge, then nuke it the next day (and the next, and the next) for a hearty, healthy, power-packed meal.

Macho Gazpacho (Powerfoods: 3)

3	large tomatoes
150 g/5½ oz	cucumber, peeled and chopped
115 g/4 oz	low-fat natural yogurt
1	teaspoon balsamic vinegar
1	teaspoon olive oil
1	teaspoon lemon juice
¼	teaspoon salt

Seed the tomatoes (cut a cross in the bottom, hold over the sink and squeeze – most of the seeds will come out of the bottom). Core and chop them into rough chunks and chuck them, along with everything else, into the blender. Purée until smooth. Serve cold.

Serves 2

Per serving: 184 cals/777 kJ, 10 g protein, 25 g carbohydrates, 5.5 g fat (1.5 g saturated), 5 g fibre, 612 mg sodium

The Beaning of Life (Powerfoods: 3)

1½	cans black beans (ideally no-salt-added), drained
120 ml/4 fl oz	low-sodium chicken stock
1	plum tomato, chopped
1	spring onion, sliced
1	tablespoon lime juice
1	teaspoon Tabasco sauce
1	teaspoon olive oil
1	tablespoon chopped fresh coriander
½	teaspoon cumin
	Salt and pepper, to taste
1	tablespoon grated reduced-fat Cheddar cheese

Dump everything except the cheese into the blender. Purée until smooth, scraping the sides if needed. Pour into bowls and microwave for 2 or 3 minutes, stirring occasionally. Top with a pinch of cheese.

Serves 4
Per serving: 198 cals/842 kJ, 15 g protein, 31 g carbohydrates,
2.5 g fat (1 g saturated), 5.5 g fibre, 253 mg sodium

Pitta Pizzas

Contrary to popular belief, pizza *is* a health food. The tomato sauce provides vitamin C and the anticancer nutrient lycopene; the cheese gives you a hit of calcium and protein; and any vegetables you toss on top bring extra helpings of vitamins, minerals and fibre.

Unfortunately, most commercial pizzas are corrupted by excess oil, fatty pepperoni and horrific mutations like 'cheese-filled crust'. Talk about turning a good thing bad!

On page 165, I've taken a closer look at the major pizza chains. But when you want a quick hit, try these home versions for the taste without suffocating your organs in pepperoni. For all of them, spread sauce evenly over pitta bread, then top with the remaining ingredients. Bake in an oven preheated to 230°C/475°F/gas 8 for 4 to 6 minutes. All serve 1.

All White Now (Powerfoods: 5)

    1 wholemeal pitta
      White sauce (stir together 60 g/2 oz low-fat soft
      cheese or ricotta cheese, 1 teaspoon olive oil,
      ¼ teaspoon dried basil or oregano)
    1 spring onion, sliced
    1 tablespoon reduced-fat mozzarella cheese
40 g/1¼ oz cooked chicken, diced; 30 g/1 oz smoked salmon,
      chopped; or 3 slices tomato

Chicken: Per serving: 411 cals/1730 kJ, 30 g protein, 44 g carbohydrates, 15 g fat (6.5 g saturated), 2 g fibre, 685 mg sodium
Salmon: Per serving: 381 cals/1603 kJ, 26 g protein, 44 g carbohydrates, 13 g fat (6 g saturated), 2 g fibre, 1216 mg sodium
Tomato: Per serving: 347 cals/1460 kJ, 19 g protein, 45 g carbohydrates, 12 g fat (6 g saturated), 2.5 g fibre, 657 mg sodium

Red Alert (Powerfoods: 3)

1 wholemeal pitta

60 ml/ 2 fl oz tomato-based pasta sauce

1 spring onion, sliced

2 tablespoons grated reduced-fat mozzarella cheese

3 frozen turkey meatballs, defrosted; 2 turkey slices, chopped; or ½ green pepper (capsicum), chopped

Meatball: Per serving: 286 cals/1215 kJ, 21 g protein, 46 g carbohydrates, 3 g fat (1 g saturated), 2 g fibre, 608 mg sodium

Turkey: Per serving: 283 cals/1200 kJ, 22 g protein, 46 g carbohydrates, 3 g fat (0.5 g saturated), 2 g fibre, 596 mg sodium

Pepper: Per serving: 228 cals/969 kJ, 8.5 g protein, 47 g carbohydrates, 2 g fat (0.5 g saturated), 3 g fibre, 578 mg sodium

The Pancho Villa (Powerfoods: 2)

1 wholemeal pitta

60 ml/2 fl oz salsa

1 teaspoon chopped fresh coriander

2 tablespoons grated reduced-fat Cheddar cheese

40 g/1¼ oz cooked chicken, diced; ¼ green or red pepper (capsicum), chopped; or ¼ avocado, chopped

Chicken: Per serving: 367 cals/1549 kJ, 28.5 g protein, 46 g carbohydrates, 8.5 g fat (4 g saturated), 2 g fibre, 287 mg sodium

Pepper: Per serving: 306 cals/1294kJ, 17.5 g protein, 48 g carbohydrates, 6 g fat (3 g saturated), 3 g fibre, 533 mg sodium

Avocado: Per serving: 389 cals/1634 kJ, 18 g protein, 47 g carbohydrates, 15 g fat (5 g saturated), 3.5 g fibre, 533 mg sodium

Chapter 7

START YOUR NIGHT RIGHT

30 Abs Diet Dinners

TYPICAL SCENARIO: for the first 10 or 12 hours of your day, your life is somebody else's, whether you're working for a boss or catering to your kids. And just about the time you finally finish feeding everybody else's needs, your stomach starts sending you signals that it's tired of being ignored.

When you work hard all day – especially if you're too busy to eat right – it makes sense that you'd want to reward yourself with a big plate of Whatever the Hell You Want, maybe washed down with a Manhattan and a couple of glasses of wine. And dinners should be a celebration of sorts: there's nothing wrong with rewarding yourself for forging through another demanding day and taking time to surround yourself with family, friends – and food.

But you can have your reward without sacrificing your health or your waistline. How well you eat at dinner is in great part determined by what you ate earlier in the day. If you fuel your body throughout the day with four smart, sensible meals and snacks, you'll find you aren't ravenously hungry the minute you walk in the door or craving the half-a-pig special at O'Bloaty's Tavern. You can, instead, enjoy a hearty – and healthy – meal, either at your favourite restaurant or at home with one of these simple recipes. Instead of using dinner as an opportunity to get drunk on fat and sweets, use it as an opportunity to pack in as many of the POWER 12 as you can.

Burgers

Burgers don't have to resemble deep-fried hockey pucks. Make yours with lean beef or turkey, grill it just the way you want it, and enjoy a protein blast that will fire up your fat-burners and stimulate muscle growth. Most supermarkets now carry wholemeal hamburger buns, so your classic 'junk-food' dinner can morph into a perfect diet food – without sacrificing taste.

The Official Abs Diet Burger (Powerfoods: 5)

1 egg
455 g/1 lb lean minced beef
40 g/1¼ oz oats
½ small onion, finely chopped
30 g/1 oz spinach, chopped
2 tablespoons grated reduced-fat Cheddar cheese
Salt and pepper

In a large bowl, whisk the egg. Add everything else, mixing it – your hands are the best tool – until well blended. Form into four patties. Put the burgers in a grill pan or non-stick frying pan over medium-high heat. Cook for 6 minutes per side or to the desired doneness.

Serves 4 (Wrap any extra burgers and freeze them for later.)

Per serving: 278 cals/1166 kJ, 30 g protein, 7 g carbohydrates, 14 g fat (6 g saturated), 1 g fibre, 182 mg sodium

Alaskan Burger (Powerfoods: 4)

1 egg (use omega-3 eggs to up the good-fat count)

1 can (418 g/14½ oz) salmon, drained

2 slices wholemeal toast, cubed

1 tablespoon ground flaxseed

Salt and pepper

Preheat oven to 190°C/375°F/gas 5. In a large bowl, break open the egg and stir. Add everything else, mixing it with your hand until well blended. Form into four patties. Bake in the oven for 20 minutes, turning once.

Serves 4

Per serving: 240 cals/1006 kJ, 25 g protein, 8 g carbohydrates, 11.5 g fat (2 g saturated), 1 g fibre, 708 mg sodium

Ciao Down Burger (Powerfoods: 2)

1 egg

455 g/1 lb minced turkey breast

2 cloves garlic, crushed

60 g/2 oz drained canned chopped tomatoes

1 teaspoon dried basil

¼ teaspoon salt

In a large bowl, whisk the egg. Add everything else, mixing it with your hand until well blended. Form into four patties. Put the patties in a grill pan or non-stick frying pan over medium-high heat. Cook for 6 minutes per side or to the desired doneness.

Serves 4

Per serving: 142 cals/598 kJ, 27 g protein, 0.5 g carbohydrates, 3 g fat (1 g saturated), 0.2 g fibre, 248 mg sodium

Chicken and Turkey

Ask a culinary adventurer to describe the flavour of any exotic dish, from frogs' legs to turtle soup to medallions of rattlesnake, and chances are you'll hear it 'tastes like chicken'.

That's not a lot of respect given to the humble chicken and its larger cousin, the turkey. But these two birds are powerful sources of lean protein and great go-to options whenever you're stuck for something to eat. Try these simple concoctions out for size, and the answer to the eternal question, 'What does it taste like?' will always be, 'Tastes like I want more.'

Faux Fried Chicken (Powerfoods: 3)

50 g/1¾ oz high-fibre bran flakes

1 egg

Tabasco sauce, to taste

2 boneless, skinless chicken breasts

Preheat oven to 180°C/350°F/gas 4. Put the cereal in a zip-top bag, seal, and pound the hell out of it. In a large bowl, whisk the egg and desired amount of Tabasco together. Dip chicken breasts in egg mixture, then roll in crushed cereal. Bake in the oven for 20 minutes.

Serves 2

Per serving: 316 cals/1336 kJ, 47 g protein, 18 g carbohydrates, 6 g fat (2 g saturated), 3 g fibre, 367 mg sodium

The Dijon Lennon (Powerfoods: 3)

2 boneless, skinless turkey breast steaks

1 teaspoon olive oil

80 ml/3 fl oz low-sodium chicken stock

1 tablespoon Dijon mustard

2 spring onions, sliced

Salt and pepper, to taste

Pound the turkey to an even thickness. Heat the oil in a non-stick frying pan over medium heat. Brown the turkey for about 3 minutes per side. Add stock, mustard, onions, salt and pepper, stirring well. Reduce heat to low. Simmer for 10 to 12 minutes.

Serves 2

Per serving: 218 cals/917 kJ, 36 g protein, 1 g carbohydrates, 8 g fat (1.5 g saturated), 0.1 g fibre, 408 mg sodium

Chicken à l'Orange (Powerfoods: 4)

1 teaspoon olive oil

2 boneless, skinless chicken breasts

3 tablespoons orange juice

1 teaspoon grated orange zest

1 tablespoon low-sodium soy sauce

¼ teaspoon ground ginger

1 spring onion, sliced

1 tablespoon flaked almonds

1 teaspoon chopped coriander

Heat the oil in a non-stick frying pan over medium heat. Add chicken and sear for 3 minutes per side. Add orange juice and zest, soy sauce and ginger, stirring to mix. Reduce heat and simmer for 5 to 6 minutes. To serve, top with the spring onion, almonds and coriander.

Serves 2

Per serving: 331 cals/1387 kJ, 45 g protein, 3.5 g carbohydrates, 15 g fat (2 g saturated), 1 g fibre, 610 mg sodium

Precooked Chicken

Precooked chicken – low in saturated fat and high in protein – is ideal for busy people. You can eat it plain, chop it up and toss it onto a salad for a quick protein boost, or cook with it. Just beware, though – in order to preserve the chicken for your ease of use, these chicken pieces are saltier than fresh, uncooked chicken.

Que Sera Quesadilla (Powerfoods: 4)

2	wholewheat tortillas
60 g/2 oz	grated reduced-fat Cheddar cheese
75 g/2½ oz	grilled chicken, diced
1	heaped tablespoon chopped fresh coriander
1	spring onion, sliced
	Salsa

Put 1 tortilla in a preheated non-stick frying pan over medium-low heat. Top with ½ of the cheese and the chicken, coriander and onion. Add the remaining cheese and top with the other tortilla, pressing down to flatten. Cook for 3 minutes, then flip and cook 3 minutes more. Serve with salsa.

Serves 1
Per serving: 524 cals/2209 kJ, 47 g protein, 50 g carbohydrates, 16 g fat (7 g saturated), 0.1 g fibre, 595 mg sodium

Gonzo Chicken (Powerfoods: 8)

115 g/4 oz	mixed green salad
60 g/2 oz	baby spinach leaves
100 g/3½ oz	chickpeas, rinsed and drained
75 g/2½ oz	cooked chicken, diced
1	tablespoon chopped pecans
1	spring onion, sliced
3	slices avocado
2	teaspoons olive oil
1½	tablespoons balsamic or red wine vinegar
	Salt and pepper, to taste

Mix leaves, chickpeas, chicken, nuts and spring onion together in a bowl. Top with avocado, oil and vinegar.

Serves 1

Per serving: 506 cals/2109 kJ, 34 g protein, 23 g carbohydrates,
31 g fat (5 g saturated), 8.5 g fibre, 156 mg sodium

It Takes Stew, Baby (Powerfoods: 5)

115 g/4 oz   baby spinach leaves, roughly torn

1   red pepper (capsicum), diced

1   clove garlic, crushed

1   teaspoon olive oil

300 g/10½ oz   canned cannellini beans, drained and rinsed

150 g/5½ oz   cooked chicken, cubed

120 ml/4 fl oz   low-sodium chicken stock

Salt and pepper, to taste

In a non-stick frying pan heated over medium-low heat, sauté the
spinach, pepper and garlic in oil for 2 minutes, turning frequently.
Add the beans and chicken. Sauté for a further 1 minute. Add stock.
Simmer for 10 minutes. Add salt and pepper to taste.

Serves 2

Per serving: 255 cals/1076 kJ, 28 g protein, 26 g carbohydrates,
5 g fat (1 g saturated), 9.5 g fibre, 1016 mg sodium

Steak

Red meat pulsates with amino acids, the breeze blocks of your
body's architecture. In fact, steak is the best natural source of
creatine, an enzyme that helps stimulate muscle growth. So
unleash your inner carnivore, and you'll unleash your abs as
well.

Fruit of Your Loins (Powerfoods: 3)

2	beef fillet steaks
1 teaspoon	olive oil
2	cloves garlic, finely chopped
¼ teaspoon	pepper
75 g/2½ oz	raspberries or blackberries
80 ml/3 fl oz	red wine
	Salt

Cook steaks in a frying pan over medium-high heat for 2 minutes per side. Remove from pan. Add the oil, sauté the garlic for 30 seconds, then add pepper, berries and wine. Return the steaks to the pan and cook for 4 to 6 minutes, or to the desired doneness. Add salt to taste.

Serves 2

Per serving: 285 cals/1196 kJ, 44 g protein, 2 g carbohydrates, 8 g fat (3 g saturated), 1 g fibre, 501 mg sodium

Sergeant Pepper (Powerfoods: 4)

170 g/6 oz	flank (skirt) steak
½	green or red pepper (capsicum), cut lengthways into strips
45 g/1½ oz	cashew nuts, chopped
2	spring onions, sliced
3 tablespoons	reduced-sodium soy sauce
	Tabasco sauce, to taste
1 teaspoon	sugar

Cut meat diagonally and across the grain into thin strips (freezing it for 20 minutes first helps a lot). Place in a large zip-top plastic bag with all other ingredients. Shake well to combine. Place in a hot frying pan over medium-high heat. Cook for 5 to 6 minutes, or until meat reaches desired doneness, turning frequently.

Serves 2

Per serving: 342 cals/1432 kJ, 36 g protein, 8 g carbohydrates, 19 g fat (5.5 g saturated), 2 g fibre, 1183 mg sodium

Steak Fa-heat-as (Powerfoods: 4)

170 g/6 oz flank (skirt) steak

1 small onion, cut into eighths

1 green or red pepper (capsicum), cut lengthways into strips

1 small jalapeño (hot chilli) pepper, cut into rings

1 teaspoon olive oil

1 tablespoon chopped fresh coriander

⅛ teaspoon ground cinnamon

¼ teaspoon ground cumin

Salt and pepper, to taste

Cut meat diagonally and across the grain into thin strips. Place in a large zip-top plastic bag with all other ingredients. Shake well to combine. Place in a hot frying pan over medium-high heat. Cook for 5 to 6 minutes, or until meat reaches desired doneness, turning frequently. Serve with four wholewheat tortillas and salsa.

Serves 2

Per serving: 478 cals/2020 kJ, 39 g protein, 59 g carbohydrates, 11 g fat (4 g saturated), 2 g fibre, 589 mg sodium

Mighty Muffins (Powerfoods: 3)

1 egg

455 g/1 lb lean minced beef

2 tablespoons balsamic vinegar

40 g/1¼ oz oats

½ small onion, finely chopped

Salt and pepper, to taste

Preheat oven to 190°C/375°F/gas 5. In a large bowl, whisk the egg. Add everything else, mixing with your hand until well blended. Divide mixture into a 6-cup non-stick muffin tin. Bake for 25 minutes.

Serves 3 (Wrap extras and freeze them for later.)

Per serving: 349 cals/1465 kJ, 41 g protein, 10 g carbohydrates, 16 g fat (6.5 g saturated), 1 g fibre, 401 mg sodium

Aztec Casserole (Powerfoods: 3)

170 g/6 oz lean minced beef

1 small onion, finely chopped

1 clove garlic, crushed

¼ teaspoon ground cumin

340 g/12 oz cooked brown rice

180 ml/6 fl oz salsa

1 tablespoon chopped coriander

2 tablespoons grated reduced-fat Cheddar cheese

Brown beef in a large non-stick frying pan over medium heat (about 3 to 4 minutes). Add onion and garlic and sauté 3 to 5 minutes or until soft. Drain the fat. Add cumin, rice, salsa and coriander, stirring to mix well. Reduce heat to low and simmer for 6 to 8 minutes. Top each serving with a tablespoon of cheese.

Serves 2

Per serving: 478 cals/2013 kJ, 31 g protein, 65 g carbohydrates, 12 g fat (5 g saturated), 2 g fibre, 167 mg sodium

One-Pot Dishes

Most of us don't mind the cooking so much as we mind the cleaning, which is where these recipes come in. Everything gets cooked in one pan, which leaves you more time for *Nip / Tuck* reruns.

Three Amigos Chilli (Powerfoods: 5)

1 tablespoon olive oil

1 small onion, finely chopped

1 small jalapeño (hot chilli) pepper, chopped

455 g/1 lb minced turkey breast

300 g/10½ oz each canned chickpeas, black beans and kidney beans, drained and rinsed

400 g/14 oz canned chopped tomatoes

400 ml/14 fl oz low-sodium chicken stock

¼ teaspoon each salt and ground cumin

⅛ teaspoon ground cinnamon

Tabasco sauce, to taste

Heat oil in a frying pan over medium-low heat. Add onion and chilli, sauté until soft (about 3 to 5 minutes). Add turkey and brown (about 5 minutes). Add beans, tomatoes with their juice, stock and spices. Stir, bring to the boil, then reduce heat and simmer for 20 minutes.

Serves 6 (Freeze leftovers and save money by taking them for lunch.)
Per serving: 175 cals/738 kJ, 22 g protein, 12 g carbohydrates, 4 g fat (0.5 g saturated), 3 g fibre, 249 mg sodium

Hot-Headed Chicken (Powerfoods: 5)

1 teaspoon olive oil

1 small onion, finely chopped

½ red pepper (capsicum), diced

1 egg

1 tablespoon reduced-sodium soy sauce

Tabasco sauce, to taste

340 g/12 oz cooked brown rice

225 g/8 oz cooked chicken, diced

Heat oil in a non-stick frying pan over medium heat. Add onion and red pepper. Sauté for 3 to 5 minutes, until onion softens. Add egg, stirring frequently. Cook for 2 to 4 minutes, until egg scrambles. Add soy sauce, Tabasco, rice and chicken. Stir and cook for a further 3 minutes, until evenly heated.

Serves 2
Per serving: 516 cals/2170 kJ, 39 g protein, 60 g carbohydrates, 15 g fat (4 g saturated), 2 g fibre, 545 mg sodium

Pot Luck of the Irish (Powerfoods: 3)

250 g/9 oz pork loin (fillet)

¼ teaspoon olive oil

1 small onion, finely chopped

½ red pepper (capsicum), diced

75 g/2½ oz cabbage, shredded

1 small tomato, chopped

80 ml/3 fl oz low-sodium chicken stock

⅛ teaspoon paprika

Salt and pepper, to taste

In a non-stick frying pan, brown the pork 2 to 3 minutes per side over medium-high heat. Remove pork. Add oil, onion and red pepper, sautéing for 3 to 5 minutes or until onion softens. Reduce heat to medium. Stir in cabbage, tomato, stock and spices. Add pork to the frying pan. Cook for a further 10 minutes, stirring occasionally.

Serves 2

Per serving: 294 cals/1235 kJ, 42 g protein, 9 g carbohydrates, 10.5 g fat (3 g saturated), 2.5 g fibre, 647 mg sodium

Seafood

To quote the culinarily confused sharks from *Finding Nemo*, fish are our friends. Fish delivers plenty of lean protein, and oily fish are packed with the omega-3 fatty acids that help control cholesterol and your appetite at the same time. To be as sleek and energetic as a dolphin, try these no-hassle recipes.

Popeye's Prawns (Powerfoods: 3)

24 large prawns, peeled and deveined

30 g/1 oz baby spinach leaves, chopped

1 teaspoon olive oil

1 clove garlic, crushed

1 teaspoon chopped fresh basil
or ½ teaspoon dried basil

Tabasco sauce, to taste

Mix all the ingredients in a large microwave-safe bowl, tossing well to coat the prawns. Microwave on high for 1 minute. Remove and toss again. Microwave for a further 1¼ minutes.

Serves 2

Per serving: 117 cals/492 kJ, 22 g protein, 1 g carbohydrates, 2.5 g fat (0.5 g saturated), 0.5 g fibre, 1607 mg sodium

The Aqua Man (Powerfoods: 3)

10 small spears asparagus, trimmed

60 g/2 oz carrots, cut into matchsticks

1 teaspoon olive oil

Juice of 1 lemon

½ teaspoon grated lemon zest

1 clove garlic, crushed

Salt and pepper, to taste

2 white fish fillets

In a small bowl, mix the vegetables with the oil, lemon juice, zest, garlic, salt and pepper. Arrange the fish in a small, shallow microwave-safe baking dish. Pour the vegetable mixture over each fillet. Cover dish tightly in cling film, pricking it a couple of times with a fork or skewer. Microwave on high for 3 to 4 minutes or until the fish flakes lightly with a fork.

Serves 2

Per serving: 148 cals/623 kJ, 25 g protein, 5 g carbohydrates, 3 g fat (0.5 g saturated), 3 g fibre, 101 mg sodium

Fish Tacos (Powerfoods: 3)

2 frozen fish fillets, Cajun- or blackened-style

4 small corn tortillas

60 g/2 oz baby spinach, chopped

4 tablespoons grated reduced-fat Cheddar cheese

Salsa

Microwave fish according to the instructions on the packet. Slice fillets into strips, then divide evenly among the four tortillas. Top with spinach, cheese and salsa to taste.

Serves 2

Per serving: 309 cals/1300 kJ, 37 g protein, 16 g carbohydrates, 11 g fat (5 g saturated), 0.5 g fibre, 352 mg sodium

Hot Pink (Powerfoods: 3)

2 90-g/3-oz pieces of fresh salmon

1½ tablespoons reduced-sodium soy sauce

1 teaspoon olive oil

Tabasco sauce, to taste

¼ teaspoon ground ginger

1 spring onion, sliced

1 teaspoon chopped fresh coriander

Place the fish on a foil-lined grill pan. Grill 4 to 5 minutes or until fish flakes with a fork. Meanwhile, mix soy sauce, olive oil, Tabasco, ginger, onion and coriander in a small microwave-safe bowl. Microwave on high for 2 minutes, stirring once. Remove fish from the grill. Transfer to a plate, then pour half the soy sauce mixture over each piece of fish.

Serves 2

Per serving: 185 cals/772 kJ, 19 g protein, 2 g carbohydrates, 11.5 g fat (2 g saturated), 0 g fibre, 991 mg sodium

The Perfect Storm (Powerfoods: 3)

2 white fish fillets

2 tablespoons mustard

1 egg, beaten

60 g/2 oz pecans, finely chopped

Honey

Preheat oven to 180°C/350°F/gas 4. Spread each fish fillet with about 1 tablespoon of mustard, then dip in beaten egg. Roll in chopped nuts. Bake in the oven for 10 to 12 minutes or until the fish flakes. When done, drizzle each fillet lightly with honey.

Serves 2

Per serving: 357 cals/1483 kJ, 28 g protein, 3 g carbohydrates, 26 g fat (3 g saturated), 1.5 g fibre, 570 mg sodium

Pasta

Legend has it that Martin Scorsese took Robert De Niro to Little Italy and directed him to eat pasta in order to balloon up for the second act of *Raging Bull*. But that doesn't mean you can't eat spaghetti and still look fighting trim. Whenever possible, opt for wholewheat versions; they'll give you gut-filling fibre and help take out a hit on your cholesterol. But with all pasta dishes, the key is to avoid fatty sauces and pile your plate high with Powerfoods.

The You-Can Noodle (Powerfoods: 3)

10 or 12 frozen turkey meatballs

400 g/14 oz canned chopped tomatoes

1 teaspoon chopped fresh basil or ½ teaspoon dried basil

1 clove garlic, crushed

115 g/4 oz wholewheat spaghetti, cooked

2 tablespoons grated reduced-fat mozzarella cheese

Defrost meatballs according to the directions on the packet. Toss with tomatoes, basil and garlic. Microwave on high for 2 minutes, stirring once. Toss with cooked pasta and top with cheese.

Serves 2

Per serving: 295 cals/1257 kJ, 43 g protein, 20 g carbohydrates, 5 g fat (2 g saturated), 3.5 g fibre, 306 mg sodium

'Alfredo, I Know It Was You . . .'(Powerfoods: 6)

1 teaspoon	olive oil
1 clove	garlic, crushed
115 g/4 oz	ricotta cheese, reduced-fat if available
60 ml/2 fl oz	skimmed milk
170 g/6 oz	canned salmon, drained
115 g/4 oz	wholewheat spaghetti, cooked
2 tablespoons	grated reduced-fat mozzarella cheese
	Salt and pepper, to taste

In a frying pan, heat oil and garlic over low-medium heat for 1 minute. Add ricotta and milk, stir, then add the salmon and simmer for 5 to 6 minutes. Thin with additional milk if needed. Pour over the cooked pasta and top with mozzarella. Add salt and pepper to taste.

Serves 2

Per serving: 360 cals/1515 kJ, 32 g protein, 17 g carbohydrates, 19 g fat (3 g saturated), 2 g fibre, 673 mg sodium

The Pesto Résistance (Powerfoods: 5)

1 tablespoon	olive oil
60 g/2 oz	walnut pieces
1 clove	garlic, crushed
115 g/4 oz	baby spinach leaves, torn
2 teaspoons	chopped fresh basil or 1 teaspoon dried basil
	Salt and pepper, to taste
115 g/4 oz	wholewheat spaghetti, cooked
2 tablespoons	grated reduced-fat mozzarella cheese

Heat oil in a non-stick frying pan over medium-low heat. Add nuts and toast for 3 to 4 minutes, stirring frequently. Add garlic, spinach, basil, salt and pepper. Cook for a further 3 to 5 minutes, turning frequently. Toss with the cooked pasta and top with mozzarella.

Serves 2

Per serving: 340 cals/1414 kJ, 14 g protein, 15 g carbohydrates, 25 g fat (3 g saturated), 4 g fibre, 209 mg sodium

Side Dishes

No matter what your main course, it's always smart to build your side dishes from the ABS DIET POWER 12 – whether it's brown rice, spinach, salad or beans. But you have many other options, as well.

The Breathalyzer (Powerfoods: 2)

1 teaspoon olive oil

1 clove garlic, crushed

170 g/6 oz baby spinach leaves, roughly torn

Heat olive oil in a frying pan over medium-high heat. Add garlic and sauté for 2 minutes. Add spinach, sautéing 3 to 5 minutes until all the leaves are wilted, turning frequently with tongs.

Serves 2

Per serving: 36 cals/149 kJ, 2.5 g protein, 1.5 g carbohydrates, 2 g fat (0.3 g saturated), 2 g fibre, 119 mg sodium

The Green Party (Powerfoods: 2)

225 g/8 oz fresh green beans, trimmed into 2.5-cm/1-in long pieces

1 heaped tablespoon flaked almonds

¼ teaspoon grated lemon zest

Salt, to taste

Juice of ½ lemon

Arrange beans, almonds, lemon zest and salt (in that order) in a steamer. Squeeze the lemon juice over the top. Steam to desired texture (3 to 5 minutes for firm beans). Add more salt to taste.

Serves 2

Per serving: 89 cals/367kJ, 4 g protein, 4 g carbohydrates, 6 g fat (0.5 g saturated), 3 g fibre, 394 mg sodium

Nuclear Orange Spud Missiles (Powerfoods: 1)

2 sweet potatoes

2 tablespoons finely chopped pecans

2 tablespoons raisins

2 teaspoons butter

Pierce potatoes with a fork. Microwave on high for 6 to 8 minutes, turning once. Cut them open and top each with 1 tablespoon pecans, 1 tablespoon raisins and 1 teaspoon butter.

Serves 2

Per serving: 287 cals/1206 kJ, 3 g protein, 38 g carbohydrates, 15 g fat (3.5 g saturated), 3 g fibre, 78 mg sodium

El El Bean (Powerfoods: 3)

150 g/5½ oz canned black beans, drained and rinsed

170 g/6 oz canned sweetcorn kernels, drained and rinsed

1 spring onion, sliced

1 teaspoon chopped fresh coriander

1 teaspoon olive oil

¼ teaspoon chilli flakes

Salt and pepper, to taste

Mix the ingredients together in a bowl.

Serves 2

Per serving: 121 cals/512 kJ, 9 g protein, 17 g carbohydrates,
2.5 g fat (0.5 g saturated), 4 g fibre, 1372 mg sodium

Jerry's Rice (Powerfoods: 2)

200 g/7 oz brown rice

low-sodium chicken stock

145 g/5 oz broccoli florets, cut uniformly to thumb tip-sized
pieces

Cook rice according to the directions on the packet, substituting
chicken stock for the recommended amount of water. Add broccoli
3–4 minutes before end of cooking time.

Serves 4

Per serving: 192 cals/814 kJ, 5 g protein, 41 g carbohydrates,
2 g fat (0.5 g saturated), 2 g fibre, 86 mg sodium

Chapter 8

SHAKE THINGS UP

27 Abs Diet Smoothies and Snacks

WE LIKE TO DRINK – whether it's beer, Coke or shots off the bartender's belly. But all drinks are not made alike – and some drinks can really sabotage your diet (or your relationship, in the case of the belly shots).

While some drinks, like sports drinks and lager, are laden with empty calories, the right drinks can jump-start your metabolism and top off your tank with a healthy dose of Powerfoods. If you've got 3 minutes to spare, you can mix up a Powerfood smoothie. Dump the ingredients in a blender, push the button, and whip up a frenzy of belly-busting nutrition.

The best thing about smoothies is their versatility. You can down a smoothie at breakfast, use it as a meal replacement at lunch, make it your late-afternoon snack to take the edge off before dinner, or have it at night as your dessert. For all recipes, first blend together any liquid ingredients (milk, yogurt, juice, etc.) and protein powder; this will help break down the grainy powder and make sure it's evenly distributed. Next, add mushy ingredients, like precooked oats and fruit, then add ice at the end. For a thicker shake, you can toss in more ice cubes; you'll add volume without the calories.

Check Your Blackberry (Powerfoods: 5)

60 g/2 oz instant oats, nuked in water

50 g/1¾ oz blackberries

2 tablespoons low-fat natural yogurt

2 teaspoons vanilla whey protein powder

1 teaspoon ground flaxseed

3 ice cubes

Makes 2 240-ml/8-fl oz servings
Per serving: 170 cals/718 kJ, 8 g protein, 27 g carbohydrates, 4 g fat (0.5 g saturated), 3 g fibre, 65 mg sodium

Choco-nana (Powerfoods: 4)

240 ml/8 fl oz skimmed chocolate milk

1 banana

2 tablespoons low-fat vanilla yogurt

1 tablespoon chopped walnuts

2 teaspoons chocolate whey protein powder

6 ice cubes

Makes 2 240-ml/8-fl oz servings
Per serving: 219 cals/922 kJ, 9 g protein, 31 g carbohydrates, 7 g fat (2 g saturated), 1 g fibre, 108 mg sodium

The Orangeman (Powerfoods: 3)

240 ml/8 fl oz skimmed milk

> 5 tablespoons orange marmalade
>
> 2 tablespoons low-fat natural yogurt
>
> 1 banana
>
> 2 teaspoons whey protein powder
>
> 6 ice cubes

Makes 2 240-ml/8-fl oz servings
Per serving: 224 cals/951 kJ, 9 g protein, 49 g carbohydrates,
1 g fat (0.5 g saturated), 1 g fibre, 138 mg sodium

Tirami-Smooth (Powerfoods: 5)

170 g/6 oz ricotta cheese, reduced-fat if available

> 2 tablespoons low-fat natural yogurt
>
> 1 tablespoon flaked almonds
>
> 2 teaspoons chocolate whey protein powder
>
> 2 teaspoons ground flaxseed
>
> ½ teaspoon finely ground coffee
>
> 6 ice cubes

Makes 2 240-ml/8-fl oz servings
Per serving: 256 cals/1073 kJ, 16 g protein, 9 g carbohydrates,
18.5 g fat (0.5 g saturated), 0.5 g fibre, 135 mg sodium

The Endless Summer (Powerfoods: 4)

60 ml/2 fl oz skimmed milk

115 g/4 oz watermelon, seeded and cubed

75 g/2½ oz strawberries

115 g/4 oz low-fat natural yogurt

2 teaspoons vanilla whey protein powder

3 ice cubes

Makes 2 240-ml/8-fl oz servings

Per serving: 87 cals/369 kJ, 6 g protein, 14 g carbohydrates, 1 g fat (0.5 g saturated), 0.5 g fibre, 92 mg sodium

Punk'd Pie (Powerfoods: 5)

115 g/4 oz canned, steamed or microwaved pumpkin

60 g/2 oz instant oats, nuked in water

30 g/1 oz chopped pecans

2 tablespoons low-fat vanilla yogurt

2 teaspoons vanilla whey protein powder

1 teaspoon ground flaxseed

3 ice cubes

Makes 2 240-ml/8-fl oz servings

Per serving: 300 cals/1259 kJ, 9 g protein, 35 g carbohydrates, 15 g fat (2 g saturated), 3 g fibre, 60 mg sodium

Lime Dancing (Powerfoods: 3)

2 tablespoons lime juice cordial

240 ml/8 fl oz skimmed milk

2 tablespoons low-fat vanilla yogurt

1 banana

2 teaspoons vanilla whey protein powder

3 ice cubes

Makes 2 240-ml/8-fl oz servings

Per serving: 156 cals/664 kJ, 8 g protein, 31 g carbohydrates, 1 g fat (0.5 g saturated), 0.5 g fibre, 108 mg sodium

Honey-Pecan Smoothie (Powerfoods: 5)

120 ml/4 fl oz skimmed milk

115 g/4 oz low-fat vanilla yogurt

30 g/1 oz chopped pecans

2 teaspoons whey protein powder

PACK SNACKS

For snacks, you can eat leftovers, smoothies or smaller portions of the ABS DIET POWER 12. Make sure each snack contains one or two Powerfoods, one of which must be protein. (Note: Dairy options count as protein, too.)

Protein options

2 teaspoons peanut butter

30 g/1 oz almonds, pecans, walnuts or peanuts

3 slices low-sodium deli cold cuts

60 g/2 oz shelled edamame (green soya beans)

Dairy options

225 g/8 oz low-fat yogurt

240 ml/8 fl oz skimmed milk or chocolate milk

1½ slices reduced-fat cheese

1 stick string cheese

Low-fat, no-salt-added cottage cheese

Low-fat yogurt smoothie

Fruit or vegetable options

30 g/1 oz raisins

Raw vegetables (celery, baby carrots, broccoli) in unlimited quantity

200 g/7 oz berries

1 teaspoon honey

2 teaspoons ground flaxseed

6 ice cubes

Makes 2 240-ml/8-fl oz servings

Per serving: 226 cals/947 kJ, 8.5 g protein, 19 g carbohydrates,
13 g fat (1 g saturated), 1 g fibre, 93 mg sodium

---

115 g/4 oz cantaloupe (orange-fleshed) melon

1 large orange

Wholegrain options

1 or 2 slices wholegrain bread

1 bowl oats or high-fibre cereal

3 wholewheat crackers

30 g/1 oz fat-free popcorn

1 granola (muesli) bar

Dessert options

As long as you're pairing them with Powerfoods (like a glass of milk),
these indulgences will add a taste of decadence to a healthy snack.

2 After Eight mints

3 bite-size Snickers or chocolate-coated Brazil nuts

60 g/2 oz reduced-fat ice cream

Desk-drawer snacks

These snacks balance complex carbs and protein. When buying energy
bars, look for one that is reasonably high in protein and fibre.

* 20 g/³⁄4 oz pumpkin seeds (3 g carbs, 1 g fibre, 5 g protein)

* SiS Go Bar (43 g carbs, 2 g fibre, 8 g protein)

* High5 Energy Bar (49 g carbs, 3 g fibre, 2 g protein)

Mango Tango (Powerfoods: 4)

90 g/3 oz mango, peeled and cubed

50 g/1¾ oz blueberries

½ banana

120 ml/4 fl oz skimmed milk

115 g/4 oz low-fat vanilla yogurt

2 teaspoons vanilla whey protein powder

3 ice cubes

Makes 2 240-ml/8-fl oz servings

*Per serving: 144 cals/614 kJ, 7 g protein, 29 g carbohydrates,
1 g fat (0.5 g saturated), 2 g fibre, 93 mg sodium*

Honey-Nut Cheery Oat (Powerfoods: 5)

60 g/2 oz instant oats, nuked in water

60 ml/2 fl oz skimmed milk

1 tablespoon peanut butter

2 teaspoons whey protein powder

1 teaspoon honey

1 teaspoon ground flaxseed

6 ice cubes

Makes 2 240-ml/8-fl oz servings

*Per serving: 223 cals/938 kJ, 9 g protein, 28 g carbohydrates,
9 g fat (2 g saturated), 3 g fibre, 80 mg sodium*

Blue Velvet (Powerfoods: 5)

120 ml/4 fl oz skimmed chocolate milk

115 g/4 oz low-fat vanilla yogurt

75 g/2½ oz blueberries

2 teaspoons chocolate whey protein powder

2 teaspoons ground flaxseed

3 ice cubes

Makes 2 240-ml/8-fl oz servings

Per serving: 139 cals/589 kJ, 7.5 g protein, 20 g carbohydrates, 3 g fat (1 g saturated), 1 g fibre, 94 mg sodium

The Peachy Keen (Powerfoods: 4)

240 ml/8 fl oz skimmed milk

2 tablespoons low-fat vanilla yogurt

115 g/4 oz frozen or canned, drained, peaches

75 g/2½ oz strawberries

⅛ teaspoon ground ginger

2 teaspoons whey protein powder

3 ice cubes

Makes 2 240-ml/8-fl oz servings

Per serving: 124 cals/528 kJ, 8 g protein, 23 g carbohydrates, 1 g fat (0.5 g saturated), 1 g fibre, 115 mg sodium

Cheesecake in a Cup (Powerfoods: 4)

170 g/6 oz ricotta cheese, reduced-fat if available

60 ml/2 fl oz skimmed milk

75 g/2½ oz blueberries

½ banana

2 teaspoons vanilla whey protein powder

6 ice cubes

Makes 2 240-ml/8-fl oz servings

Per serving: 208 cals/873 kJ, 13 g protein, 14 g carbohydrates, 12 g fat (0.1 g saturated), 1.5 g fibre, 113 mg sodium

Juicy Fruit Juice (Powerfoods: 4)

1 banana

75 g/2½ oz strawberries

120 ml/4 fl oz skimmed milk

2 tablespoons low-fat vanilla yogurt

80 ml/3 fl oz orange juice

2 teaspoons vanilla whey protein powder

3 ice cubes

Makes 2 240-ml/8-fl oz servings

Per serving: 145 cals/614 kJ, 6.5 g protein, 30 g carbohydrates, 1 g fat (0.5 g saturated), 1 g fibre, 87 mg sodium

Chocolate Factory (Powerfoods: 5)

240 ml/8 fl oz skimmed chocolate milk

2 tablespoons low-fat natural yogurt

2 tablespoons peanut butter

2 teaspoons chocolate whey protein powder

2 teaspoons ground flaxseed

6 ice cubes

Makes 2 240-ml/8-fl oz servings

Per serving: 259 cals/1085 kJ, 14 g protein, 19 g carbohydrates, 14 g fat (4 g saturated), 1 g fibre, 186 mg sodium

The Chocolate Latte (Powerfoods: 4)

120 ml/4 fl oz skimmed chocolate milk

115 g/4 oz low-fat natural yogurt

½ banana

1 tablespoon peanut butter

½ teaspoon finely ground coffee

2 teaspoons chocolate whey protein powder

6 ice cubes

Makes 2 240-ml/8-fl oz servings

*Per serving: 172 cals/722 kJ, 9.5 g protein, 20 g carbohydrates,
6 g fat (2 g saturated), 1 g fibre, 137 mg sodium*

Abs Diet Trail Mix (Powerfoods: 4)

A ready-made power snack is an effective one: it gives you something
to reach for when you're hungry, and it gives you good ingredients
without guilt. Make this trail mix on the weekend, then keep stashes on
hand at work and at home.

150 g/5½ oz whole almonds

100 g/3½ oz pecan halves

30 g/1 oz plain oats

Cooking spray

2 tablespoons honey

½ teaspoon ground cinnamon

115 g/4 oz dried cranberries

200 g/7 oz dried apricots

*Preheat oven to 180°C/350°F/gas 4. Place nuts and oats in a bowl
and spray evenly with cooking spray (about 3 shots). Drizzle with
1 tablespoon honey and add cinnamon, stirring to coat. Spread nut
mixture evenly on a baking tray and toast for 15 minutes, stirring
occasionally. Once it's cooled, stir in the second tablespoon of honey
and mix in the dried fruit. Divide into 50-g/1¾-oz servings and place
each in a zip-top bag.*

Makes 9 to 10 servings

*Per serving: 274 cals/1144 kJ, 6 g protein, 24 g carbohydrates,
18 g fat (1.5 g saturated), 4 g fibre, 14 mg sodium*

The Cinnamon Girl (Powerfoods: 3)

60 g/2 oz instant oats, nuked in water

2 tablespoons low-fat vanilla yogurt

1 teaspoon honey

1 teaspoon ground flaxseed

⅛ teaspoon ground cinnamon

6 ice cubes

Makes 2 240-ml/8-fl oz servings
Per serving: 171 cals/726kJ, 5 g protein, 30 g carbohydrates,
4 g fat (1 g saturated), 2 g fibre, 30 mg sodium

Peach Holiday (Powerfoods: 3)

180 ml/6 fl oz skimmed milk

170 g/6 oz frozen or canned, drained, peaches

2 tablespoons low-fat natural yogurt

2 teaspoons vanilla whey protein powder

6 ice cubes

Makes 2 240-ml/8-fl oz servings
Per serving: 102 cals/431 kJ, 7 g protein, 18 g carbohydrates,
1 g fat (0.5 g saturated), 1 g fibre, 111 mg sodium

Mint Chocolate Morning (Powerfoods: 3)

180 ml/6 fl oz skimmed chocolate milk

115 g/4 oz low-fat vanilla yogurt

2 teaspoons chocolate whey protein powder

1 Peppermint Pattie or 5 After Eight Mints, frozen

2 teaspoons ground flaxseed

3 ice cubes

Makes 2 240-ml/8-fl oz servings
Per serving: 215 cals/911 kJ, 9 g protein, 31 g carbohydrates,
7 g fat (3 g saturated), 0.5 g fibre, 120 mg sodium

The Hawaiian Five-O (Powerfoods: 4)

180 ml/6 fl oz skimmed milk

2 tablespoons low-fat natural yogurt

3 tablespoons orange marmalade

½ banana

40 g/1¼ oz strawberries

45 g/1½ oz ripe mango, cubed

2 teaspoons vanilla whey protein powder

3 ice cubes

Makes 2 240-ml/8-fl oz servings
Per serving: 189 cals/804 kJ, 8 g protein, 40 g carbohydrates,
1 g fat (0.5 g saturated), 1 g fibre, 121 mg sodium

The New Zealander (Powerfoods: 4)

240 ml/8 fl oz skimmed milk

2 tablespoons low-fat natural yogurt

1 medium peeled kiwifruit

75 g/2½ oz strawberries

2 teaspoons vanilla whey protein powder

3 ice cubes

Makes 2 240-ml/8-fl oz servings
Per serving: 103 cals/436 kJ, 9 g protein, 16 g carbohydrates,
1 g fat (0.5 g saturated), 1 g fibre, 117 mg sodium

The Almond Hammer (Powerfoods: 5)

120 ml/4 fl oz skimmed milk

115 g/4 oz low-fat vanilla yogurt

30 g/1 oz flaked almonds

2 teaspoons chocolate whey protein powder

1 teaspoon honey

1 teaspoon ground flaxseed

6 ice cubes

Makes 2 240-ml/8-fl oz servings

Per serving: 203 cals/853 kJ, 10 g protein, 20 g carbohydrates, 10 g fat (1 g saturated), 1 g fibre, 94 mg sodium

The Nutty Professor (Powerfoods: 5)

240 ml/8 fl oz skimmed chocolate milk

2 tablespoons low-fat vanilla yogurt

1 tablespoon orange marmalade

½ banana

1 tablespoon flaked almonds

2 teaspoons chocolate whey protein powder

2 teaspoons ground flaxseed

6 ice cubes

Makes 2 240-ml/8-fl oz servings

Per serving: 247 cals/1045 kJ, 10 g protein, 34 g carbohydrates, 8 g fat (2 g saturated), 1 g fibre, 117 mg sodium

The Neapolitan (Powerfoods: 5)

180 ml/6 fl oz skimmed chocolate milk

115 g/4 oz low-fat vanilla yogurt

115 g/4 oz strawberries, sliced

1 teaspoon ground flaxseed

2 teaspoons vanilla whey protein powder

3 ice cubes

Makes 2 240-ml/8-fl oz servings

Per serving: 125 cals/530 kJ, 8 g protein, 20 g carbohydrates,
2 g fat (0.5 g saturated), 1 g fibre, 109 mg sodium

The Whey-Too-Good Smoothie (Powerfoods: 6)

170 g/6 oz ricotta cheese, reduced-fat if available

180 ml/6 fl oz skimmed chocolate milk

30 g/1 oz pecans, chopped

½ banana

2 tablespoons low-fat vanilla yogurt

2 teaspoons ground flaxseed

2 teaspoons chocolate whey protein powder

6 ice cubes

Makes 2 240-ml/8-fl oz servings

Per serving: 408 cals/1408 kJ, 19 g protein, 27 g carbohydrates,
26 g fat (2 g saturated), 1 g fibre, 167 mg sodium

Abs Diet Sundae Parfait (Powerfoods: 3)

Yep, it's still a diet. The ice cream gives you calcium and protein with only a modest amount of fat and refined sugar. Indulge and enjoy!

120 ml/4 fl oz reduced-fat chocolate or vanilla ice cream

30 g/1 oz berries of your choice, slightly crushed

1 tablespoon chopped nuts of your choice

Starting with the ice cream, layer the ingredients in a small bowl.

Makes 1 serving

Per serving: 200 cals/861 kJ, 4 g protein, 17 g carbohydrates,
14 g fat (1 g saturated), 1.5 g fibre, 2 mg sodium

Chapter 9

EATING OUT, EATING RIGHT

The Abs Diet Restaurant Survival Guide

Eating out in a restaurant can be exciting, tempting, arousing ... dangerous. Here's this seductive menu in front of you – pictures and descriptions of creamy pasta, juicy burgers, cheese-drenched potato skins. They're looking at you. They're daring you. They're whispering in your ear with soft, slow, raspy voices: 'Order meeeeeee.'

So you – a person of dignity and restraint, a person with serious goals and a desire to change your body – now have to decide. Do you give in to temptation? You know what's right – what's good for you – but the temptations are crying out to you: the smells, the specials, the free bread, the 'save room for Death by Chocolate' sales pitches. Oh, just this once won't hurt ...

No, it won't. But you're going to find yourself in restaurants again and again, still facing the same choices, still being lured by the same temptations. What do you do? It's simple: look for the Powerfoods. And pull out your copy of *The Abs Diet Eat Right Every Time Guide.*

See, you don't have to sacrifice flavour to eat healthily, and you don't have to deny yourself a night out on the town. You just have to know which menu options deliver the most nutrition with the least number of empty calories and bad-for-you ingredients. To help you through the decision-making process, I've compiled a compendium of the major chain outlets and types of restaurant, with the best and the worst choices each of them has to offer.

Fast-Food Outlets

You've probably already figured out that the grilled-chicken sandwich is the default option when you don't know what else to order. But even the greasiest of junk food Valhallas offers more healthy choices than you might suspect. And even if nothing on the menu qualifies as a health food, you can still cut down on empty calories and saturated fat by ordering smartly. The goal is to stick to the plan, not bore yourself off it. One fast-food burger now and then won't kill you. Just beware of special sauces, dips and salad dressings: they're often loaded with calories and fat. Stick to ketchup, mustard or barbecue sauce. And when given the choice, a second burger is usually better than the side of fries.

Burger King (Breakfast)

ABS DIET ENDORSEMENTS:

Bacon Roll 294 calories/1235 kJ, 12 g fat, 1003 mg sodium

THE LESSER OF TWO EVILS

Eat this: *Bacon & Egg Breakfast Sandwich* 332 calories/1394 kJ, 15 g fat, 875 mg sodium	**Not that:** *Ultimate Breakfast Sandwich* 514 calories/2159 kJ, 30 g fat, 1490 mg sodium

Burger King/Hungry Jack's (Lunch & Dinner)
ABS DIET ENDORSEMENTS:

LA Flame-Grilled Chicken Salad with French Dressing 133 calories/559 kJ, 2 g fat, 611 mg sodium

Flamegrilled Chicken Sandwich 284 calories/1193 kJ, 7 g fat, 928 mg sodium

Hamburger 296 calories/1243 kJ, 12 g fat, 559 mg sodium

Piri Piri Chicken Baguette 397 calories/1667 kJ, 9 g fat, 1257 mg sodium

THE LESSER OF TWO EVILS

Eat this: *Small French Fries* 206 calories/865 kJ, 10 g fat, 539 mg sodium	**Not that:** *Large French Fries* 395 calories/1659 kJ, 20 g fat, 1034 mg sodium
Eat this: *Whopper Junior* 363 calories/1525 kJ, 19 g fat, 520 mg sodium	**Not that:** *Whopper* 614 calories/2579 kJ, 34 g fat, 908 mg sodium
Eat this: *Jacket Potato with Baked Beans* 602 calories/2528 kJ, 1 g fat, 686 mg sodium	**Not that:** *Jacket Potato with Cheese* 821 calories/3448 kJ, 28 g fat, 3086 mg sodium
Eat this: *Cajun Chicken Baguette* 412 calories/1730 kJ, 12 g fat, 1332 mg sodium	**Not that:** *Classic Cheese Burger Baguette* 574 calories/2411 kJ, 25 g fat, 1459 mg sodium

Kentucky Fried Chicken
ABS DIET ENDORSEMENTS:

Popcorn Crispy Strips (regular) 113 calories/475 kJ, 6 g fat, 400 mg sodium

Original Chicken Salad with French Dressing 299 calories/1256 kJ, 12 g fat, 1200 mg sodium

THE LESSER OF TWO EVILS

Eat this: *Fillet Burger* 409 calories/1718 kJ, 17 g fat, 900 mg sodium

Not that: *Tower Burger* 575 calories/2415 kJ, 28 g fat, 1500 mg sodium

Eat this: *Colonel's Meal (2 pieces Original Recipe chicken, regular fries, diet drink)* 527 calories/2213 kJ, 29 g fat, 500 mg sodium

Not that: *Combo Meal (2 pieces Original Recipe chicken, regular fries, BBQ beans, coleslaw, gravy, corn cobette, diet drink)* 911 calories/3826 kJ, 50 g fat, 1900 mg sodium

McDonald's (Breakfast)
ABS DIET ENDORSEMENTS:

Oatso Simple with jam 246 calories/1033 kJ, 5 g fat, 80 mg sodium

Egg McMuffin 281 calories/1180 kJ, 13 g fat, 500 mg sodium

Bagel with Light Philadelphia 318 calories/1336 kJ, 6 g fat, 680 mg sodium

Breakfast Bagel Bacon, Lettuce and Tomato 355 calories/1491 kJ, 8 g fat, 880 mg sodium

THE LESSER OF TWO EVILS

Eat this: *Bacon & Egg McMuffin* 346 calories/1453 kJ, 18 g fat, 800 mg sodium

Not that: *Breakfast Bagel Bacon, Egg and Cheese* 544 calories/2284 kJ, 24 g fat, 1360 mg sodium

Eat this: *Pancakes and syrup* 532 calories/2234 kJ, 16 g fat, 200 mg sodium

Not that: *Pancakes and sausage* 678 calories/2848 kJ, 28 g fat, 500 mg sodium

Eat this: *McBacon Roll* 349 calories/1466 kJ, 14 g fat, 1000 mg sodium

Not that: *Big Breakfast Bun* 571 calories/2398 kJ, 32 g fat, 1400 mg sodium

McDonald's (Lunch & Dinner)

ABS DIET ENDORSEMENTS:

Chicken McNuggets (4) 141 calories/592 kJ, 9 g fat, 176 mg sodium

Hamburger 253 calories/1063 kJ, 8 g fat, 476 mg sodium

Grilled Chicken Flatbread 310 calories/1302 kJ, 4 g fat, 840 mg sodium

Fruit and Yogurt 150 calories/630 kJ, 3 g fat, 200 mg sodium

THE LESSER OF TWO EVILS

Eat this: *Bacon cheeseburger* 360 calories/1512 kJ, 16 g fat, 580 mg sodium	**Not that:** *Big Mac* 493 calories/2070 kJ, 23 g fat, 900 mg sodium
Eat this: *Regular Fries* 206 calories/865 kJ, 7 g fat, 192 mg sodium	**Not that:** *Large Fries* 412 calories/1730 kJ, 18 g fat, 312 mg sodium
Eat this: *Grilled Chicken Ranch Salad without dressing* 258 calories/1084 kJ, 13 g fat, 840 mg sodium	**Not that:** *Chicken Caesar Salad with dressing and croutons* 452 calories/1898 kJ, 22 g fat, 1720 mg sodium
Eat this: *Low-fat Carrot Cake Muffin* 360 calories/1512 kJ, 4 g fat, 560 mg sodium	**Not that:** *Large Chocolate Donut* 336 calories/1411 kJ, 16 g fat, 500 mg sodium
Drink this: *Regular semi-skimmed milk* 124 calories/521 kJ, 4 g fat, 52 mg sodium	**Not that:** *Regular Strawberry Milkshake* 395 calories/1659 kJ, 10 g fat, trace sodium

Fish and Chip Shops
ABS DIET ENDORSEMENTS:

Large fried fish (batter removed) 230 calories/966 kJ, 6 g fat, 380 mg sodium

Mushy peas 105 calories/442 kJ, 1 g fat, 442 mg sodium

THE LESSER OF TWO EVILS

Eat this: *Medium fried fish (batter removed)* 200 calories/840 kJ, 5 g fat, 320 mg sodium	**Not that:** *Fish in batter (medium)* 445 calories/1869 kJ, 28 g fat, 288 mg sodium
Eat this: *Mushy peas* 105 calories/442 kJ, 1 g fat, 442 mg sodium	**Not that:** *Chips* 265 calories/1113 kJ, 29 g fat, 1000 mg sodium
Eat this: *Fishcake* 218 calories/911 kJ, 13 g fat, 510 mg sodium	**Not that:** *Sausage in batter* 434 calories/1822 kJ, 35 g fat, 1286 mg sodium

Kebab Shops
ABS DIET ENDORSEMENTS:

Chicken kebab in pitta with salad 337 calories/1432 kJ, 3 g fat, 375 mg sodium

THE LESSER OF TWO EVILS

Eat this: *Shish kebab in pitta with salad* 356 calories/1497 kJ, 9 g fat, 759 mg sodium	**Not that:** *Doner kebab in pitta with salad* 586 calories/2463 kJ, 37 g fat, 1265 mg sodium

At the Stadium

I'm a big fan of smuggling your own food into sporting events, concerts and the like: it makes healthy eating easier, it makes you feel like a little bit of a rebel, and it avoids the humiliation of queueing for an hour to pay £250 for one hot dog. But if you can't or won't smuggle a peanut butter sandwich in your underwear, you can still grab a handful of Powerfoods.

ABS DIET ENDORSEMENTS:

Hot dog (Frankfurter sausage in roll) 256 calories/1071 kJ, 14 g fat, 684 mg sodium

Popcorn (salted) (50 g bag) 297 calories/1234 kJ, 21 g fat, 1500 mg sodium

Roasted peanuts in shells, unsalted (90 g/3 oz) 510 calories/2135 kJ, 37 g fat, 3 mg sodium

THE LESSER OF TWO EVILS

Eat this: *Medium baked potato with butter* 319 calories/1352 kJ, 9 g fat, 82 mg sodium	**Not that:** *Hot chips* 420 calories/1761 kJ, 16 g fat, 465 mg sodium
Eat this: *Hot dog (Frankfurter sausage in roll)* 256 calories/1071 kJ, 14 g fat, 684 mg sodium	**Not that:** *Large sausage roll* 692 calories/2878 kJ, 53 g fat, 740 mg sodium
Eat this: *Chicken pie* 461 calories/1923 kJ, 25 g fat, 688 mg sodium	**Not that:** *Steak and kidney pie* 517 calories/2158 kJ, 34 g fat, 816 mg sodium
Eat this: *Hog roast in roll* 333 calories/1401 kJ, 12 g fat, 324 mg sodium	**Not that:** *Cornish pasty* 414 calories/1731 kJ, 25 g fat, 620 mg sodium

Eat this: *Steak sandwich (no onions)* 667 calories/2835 kJ, 8 g fat, 1294 mg sodium

Not that: *Burger and chips* 922 calories/3868 kJ, 37 g fat, 781 mg sodium

Sandwich Shops

Always start with building the right base: wholemeal bread if they have it (rye is also a good choice because it has nearly as much fibre). Then make smart choices – reduced-fat cheese (go easy on it if all they have is full-fat cheese); no fatty, salty cured cold cuts like pepperoni or salami; and top it with tomatoes and all the greens that bun can hold. And don't always trust the salads; many are loaded with saturated fats hiding in bacon pieces, croutons and goopy dressings.

ABS DIET ENDORSEMENT:

Chicken salad sandwich (no mayo) 315 calories/1330 kJ, 9.5 g fat, 594 mg sodium

Ham salad sandwich (no mayo) 300 calories/1260 kJ, 8 g fat, 1069 mg sodium

Fresh fruit salad 90 calories/378 kJ, 0.1 g fat, 5 mg sodium

THE LESSER OF TWO EVILS

Eat this: *Tuna mayonnaise sandwich* 427 calories/1793 kJ, 19 g fat, 889 mg sodium

Not that: *Cheddar cheese and pickle sandwich* 522 calories/2192 kJ, 27 g fat, 1355 mg sodium

Eat this: *Mozzarella and tomato panini* 485 calories/2048 kJ, 14 g fat, 998 mg sodium

Not that: *Ham and cheese panini* 627 calories/2637 kJ, 24 g fat, 1589 mg sodium

Eat this: *Tomato soup* 100 calories/420 kJ, 2 g fat, 500 mg sodium

Not that: *50 g potato crisps (chips)* 260 calories/1507 kJ, 18 g fat, 300 mg sodium

Choose this: No butter or spread 0 calories/0 kJ, 0 g fat, 0 mg sodium	**Not that:** Butter or spread on sandwich 118 calories/484 kJ, 13 g fat, 129 mg sodium

Pret a Manger

ABS DIET ENDORSEMENTS:

Crayfish Salad Bowl 149 calories/626 kJ, 6 g fat, 1312 mg sodium

Chicken Salad Mayo Frais Sandwich 334 calories/1403 kJ, 9 g fat, 939 mg sodium

Fresh Herb Chicken Sandwich (no mayo) 341 calories/1432 kJ, 9 g fat, 1094 mg sodium

Deluxe Sushi 522 calories/2192 kJ, 8.5 g fat, 760 mg sodium

THE LESSER OF TWO EVILS

Eat this: Slim Pret Chicken & Avocado Sandwich 260 calories/ 1092 kJ, 16 g fat, 376 mg sodium	**Not that:** Chicken & Avocado Salad Sandwich 518 calories/2177 kJ, 32 g fat, 763 mg sodium
Eat this: Big Roast Beef Sandwich 424 calories/1781 kJ, 13 g fat, 1378 mg sodium	**Not that:** Chicken Caesar Sandwich 477 calories/2003 kJ, 25 g fat, 837 mg sodium
Eat this: Pretzel 371 calories/ 1558 kJ, 8 g fat, 720 mg sodium	**Not that:** Cinnamon & Raisin Danish 408 calories/1714 kJ, 28 g fat, 300 mg sodium
Eat this: Fresh Fruit Salad 55 calories/229 kJ, 0.2 g fat, 0 mg sodium	**Not that:** Carrot Cake with Cream Cheese topping 402 calories/ 1680 kJ, 22 g fat, 335 mg sodium

Subway

ABS DIET ENDORSEMENTS:

Grilled Chicken Salad (no dressing) **146** calories/316 kJ, 0.5 g fat, 363 mg sodium

Turkey Breast Wrap **157** calories/659 kJ, 3.5 g fat, 1410 mg sodium

Deli Style Savoury Turkey Breast Sandwich **236** calories/991 kJ, 3 g fat, 790 mg sodium

6-inch sandwich <6 g fat Roast Beef **283** calories/1189 kJ, 4 g fat, 820 mg sodium

6-inch sandwich <6 g fat Roasted Chicken **304** calories/1277 kJ, 5 g fat, 940 mg sodium

THE LESSER OF TWO EVILS

Eat this: *Grilled Chicken Salad (no dressing)* 146 calories/316 kJ, 0.5 g fat, 363 mg sodium	**Not that:** *Tuna Salad* 363 calories/1525 kJ, 29 g fat, 607 mg sodium
Eat this: *6-inch Cheese Steak hot sandwich* 330 calories/1386 kJ, 9 g fat, 1290 mg sodium	**Not that:** *6-inch Meatball Marinara hot sandwich* 441 calories/1852 kJ, 18 g fat, 1500 mg sodium
Eat this: *6-inch Turkey Breast, Ham & Bacon Melt hot sandwich* 350 calories/1470 kJ, 10 g fat, 1460 mg sodium	**Not that:** *Turkey Bacon Melt wrap with chipotle sauce* 386 calories/1621 kJ, 23 g fat, 1960 mg sodium
Eat this: *Oatmeal Raisin Cookie* 193 calories/810 kJ, 8 g fat, 120 mg sodium	**Not that:** *Chocolate Chip Cookie* 218 calories/916 kJ, 11 g fat, 80 mg sodium

Breakfast Places

I can't emphasize enough the importance of eating the moment you wake up. They call it 'breakfast' for a reason – you've been fasting for the past 8 to 10 hours, and your body needs fuel. Eating immediately jump-starts your metabolism and starts you on your daily quest to turn fat into muscle. On the other hand, if you skip breakfast, even for a few hours, you signal your body to begin breaking down muscle for fuel. That's right: every minute you wait between waking and eating is a minute more of muscle loss.

That said, sometimes the fastest way to add fuel to the fire is to swing by one of these joints (especially on those mornings where you wake up somewhere . . . unusual). As a rule, make sure they don't put full-fat milk in your coffee, ask for wholemeal toast and never buy a pastry that's bigger than your head. In fact, if there's one food category I would ban if I could, it's pastries and doughnuts – or, as they're known by their technical, scientific name, 'empty sugar calories fried in lard'.

Breakfast Café

ABS DIET ENDORSEMENTS:

2 poached eggs on 2 slices toast (no butter) 275 calories/ 1158 kJ, 12 g fat, 410 mg sodium

Baked beans on 2 slices toast (no butter) 288 calories/1220 kJ, 2 g fat, 1277 mg sodium

Wholemeal toast with polyunsaturated spread (per slice) 301 calories/1262 kJ, 17 g fat, 1277 mg sodium

Cornflakes and semi-skimmed milk 170 calories/724 kJ, 2 g fat, 354 mg sodium

THE LESSER OF TWO EVILS

Eat this: *2-egg plain omelette* 195 calories/808 kJ, 17 g fat, 1024 mg sodium	**Not that:** *2-egg cheese omelette* 339 calories/1401 kJ, 29 g fat, 1151 mg sodium
Eat this: *2 rashers bacon, mushrooms, tomatoes and baked beans* 448 calories/1867 kJ, 27 g fat, 2295 mg sodium	**Not that:** *2 rashers bacon, sausage, black pudding, fried bread, fried egg* 877 calories/3650 kJ, 64 g fat, 3087 mg sodium

Coffee Shops (e.g. Costa Coffee, Coffee Club, Coffee Republic, Gloria Jean's, Starbucks)

ABS DIET ENDORSEMENTS:

Café americano or espresso 10–15 calories/42–63 kJ, 0 g fat, 0 mg sodium

Tall skinny cappuccino 83 calories/349 kJ, 0.5 g fat, 114 mg sodium

Biscotti (3 small) 101 calories/425 kJ, 3 g fat, 85 mg sodium

Skinny peach & raspberry muffin 286 calories/1202 kJ, 4.5 g fat, 421 mg sodium

THE LESSER OF TWO EVILS

Eat this: *Plain croissant* 229 calories/955 kJ, 14 g fat, 256 mg sodium	**Not that:** *Almond croissant* 481 calories/2009 kJ, 30 g fat, 425 mg sodium
Eat this: *Pain au chocolat* 241 calories/1007 kJ, 14 g fat, 270 mg sodium	**Not that:** *Raisin Danish* 360 calories/1513 kJ, 17 g fat, 375 mg sodium

Eat this: *Apple muffin* 426 calories/1790 kJ, 24 g fat, 44 mg sodium

Not that: *Double chocolate muffin* 567 calories/2360 kJ, 34 g fat, 452 mg sodium

---

Eat this: *Brownie* 300 calories/1206 kJ, 15 g fat, 168 mg sodium

Not that: *Chocolate cheesecake* 723 calories/3015 kJ, 50 g fat, 311 mg sodium

---

Eat this: *Chicken wrap* 336 calories/1405 kJ, 8 g fat, 1600 mg sodium

Not that: *Prawn Caesar wrap* 572 calories/2392 kJ, 32 g fat, 3900 mg sodium

---

Eat this: *Iced tea* 24 calories/102 kJ, 0 g fat, 15 mg sodium

Not that: *Iced coffee* 240 calories/1108 kJ, 10 g fat, 74 mg sodium

---

Bakery

ABS DIET ENDORSEMENTS:

Chocolate mini swiss roll 84 calories/355 kJ, 3 g fat, 87 mg sodium

Small iced cake 102 calories/429 kJ, 4 g fat, 65 mg sodium

Tea cake 148 calories/625 kJ, 4 g fat, 158 mg sodium

Fruit scone 158 calories/667 kJ, 4 g fat, 308 mg sodium

THE LESSER OF TWO EVILS

Eat this: *Fruit scone* 158 calories/667 kJ, 4 g fat, 308 mg sodium

Not that: *Jam doughnut* 235 calories/990 kJ, 10 g fat, 126 mg sodium

---

Eat this: *Fresh cream meringue* 132 calories/550 kJ, 8 g fat, 16 mg sodium

Not that: *Fresh cream millefeuille (puff pastry slice)* 248 calories/1037 kJ, 13 g fat, 60 mg sodium

Sit-Down Restaurants

Here's the big secret about those casual-dinner restaurants: they're really all the same. Sure, there are some slight variations, but a sirloin is a sirloin is a sirloin; maybe one place offers it in a 225 g/8 oz cut while another in 285 g/10 oz, but the meat remains the same. So even though these recommendations are not keyed to a specific restaurant, you can use them anywhere.

Steakhouses and casual restaurants (e.g. Hard Rock Café, TGI Friday)

ABS DIET ENDORSEMENTS:

Grilled chicken breast – no skin (170 g/6 oz) 251 calories/1057 kJ, 4 g fat, 93 mg sodium

Grilled salmon steak (170 g/6 oz) 365 calories/1535 kJ, 23 g fat, 92 mg sodium

Fillet steak (225 g/8 oz) 398 calories/1671 kJ, 13 g fat, 166 mg sodium

Steamed mixed vegetables or side salad with no dressing 63 calories/270 kJ, 0.5 g fat, 144 mg sodium

THE LESSER OF TWO EVILS

Eat this: *Chunky chips* 409 calories/1720 kJ, 20 g fat, 43 mg sodium	**Not that:** *French fries* 546 calories/2293 kJ, 32 g fat, 145 mg sodium
Eat this: *Corn on the cob (no butter)* 111 calories/470 kJ, 2 g fat, 1 mg sodium	**Not that:** *Garlic mushrooms* 140 calories/579 kJ, 14 g fat, 108 mg sodium

Eat this: *Bruschetta with tomato and basil* 446 calories/1888 kJ, 13 g fat, 739 mg sodium

Not that: *Barbecue chicken wings with sour cream dip* 728 calories/3033 kJ, 52 g fat, 945 mg sodium

---

Eat this: *Pavlova with cream and fresh fruit* 288 calories/1210 kJ, 13 g fat, 4 mg sodium

Not that: *Fruit pie with cream* 430 calories/1796 kJ, 20 g fat, 292 mg sodium

---

Bistros and gastropubs

ABS DIET ENDORSEMENT:

Mixed olives 103 calories/422 kJ, 11 g fat, 2250 mg sodium

Beef bourguignonne 244 calories/1022 kJ, 13 g fat, 694 mg sodium

Chargrilled tuna with tomato salsa 373 calories/1570 kJ, 13 g fat, 106 mg sodium

NUTRITIONAL DETECTIVE WORK

Food labels are all well and good when you're cooking for yourself, but what about those occasional nights (OK, endless stream of nights) when dinner is dished up by some pimply-faced kid with a paper hat and a bored expression? How do you know what, exactly, is in that paper-and-polystyrene-wrapped monstrosity you're eating? In the land of 'special sauces' and 'secret recipes', sussing out the nutritional realities of your favourite fast foods can take a little detective work.

If the greasy floor beneath your feet is that of a national fast-food joint, the answers may be pretty easy to come by. Many fast-food restaurants post complete nutritional information on their websites. Many will also have posters hanging in some dim corner of the restaurant, if you're willing to search. Be aware of two caveats: firstly, these menus may change, so you need to make sure what you're ordering is what they've posted. Secondly, watch out for serving size and extra ingredients: at

THE LESSER OF TWO EVILS

Eat this: *Butternut squash soup* 123 calories/519 kJ, 0.5 g fat, 1260 mg sodium	**Not that:** *Deep-fried Camembert with cranberry sauce* 506 calories/2104 kJ, 39 g fat, 552 mg sodium
Eat this: *Chicken noodle salad with chilli dressing* 360 calories/1519 kJ, 2 g fat, 516 mg sodium	**Not that:** *Chargrilled artichoke and pesto pasta salad* 789 calories/3338 kJ, 34 g fat, 4680 mg sodium
Eat this: *Moules and frites* 503 calories/2124 kJ, 17 g fat, 814 mg sodium	**Not that:** *Sausages, mustard mash and gravy* 650 calories/2705 kJ, 41 g fat, 2019 mg sodium
Eat this: *Baked cod with lemon butter* 248 calories/1044 kJ, 10 g fat, 657 mg sodium	**Not that:** *Thai salmon fish cakes* 436 calories/1822 kJ, 27 g fat, 1020 mg sodium

some chains, the numbers for the 'healthy' salad don't include the fried bacon pieces that come on top. Others give you the calorie count for a serving of their dressing, but the package that comes with the salad can be two or even three servings, not one.

Chain restaurants that feature actual menus and waiters are a mixed bag. Some deserve a round of applause for providing complete nutritional information on their websites. Others deserve jeers for refusing to give us a nutritional breakdown of some of their foods, even when I called their corporate headquarters and harassed them.

So check your favourite restaurant's website. Even if they only list total calories, that's enough to make an informed decision – when you read that a starter of deep-fried mushrooms has 600 calories/2520 kJ, you can pretty much figure the meal should only be administered under a cardiologist's care. If you can't find the information you want on the web, call their customer service line. They might be able to email or fax it to you. And if that's not an option, well, tell them you want it to be.

Eat this: *New potatoes* 131 calories/562 kJ, 0.5 g fat, 16 mg sodium

Not that: *Mustard mashed potato* 208 calories/878 kJ, 9 g fat, 86 mg sodium

---

Eat this: *Pear poached in red wine with ice cream* 303 calories/1273 kJ, 7 g fat, 59 mg sodium

Not that: *Sticky toffee pudding with cream* 508 calories/2128 kJ, 21 g fat, 400 mg sodium

---

Italian Restaurants

ABS DIET ENDORSEMENTS:

Minestrone soup 93 calories/396 kJ, 1.5 g fat, 906 mg sodium

Mozzarella, tomato and rocket salad 229 calories/954 kJ, 17 g fat, 324 mg sodium

Penne arrabbiata 437 calories/1845 kJ, 9 g fat, 79 mg sodium

THE LESSER OF TWO EVILS

Eat this: *Prawns in garlic and chilli* 234 calories/969 kJ, 21 g fat, 815 mg sodium

Not that: *Garlic mushrooms and bruschetta* 495 calories/2071 kJ, 31 g fat, 715 mg sodium

---

Eat this: *Spaghetti with meatballs* 404 calories/1704 kJ, 14 g fat, 468 mg sodium

Not that: *Tagliatelle with ham, cheese and mushroom sauce* 555 calories/2336 kJ, 28 g fat, 1360 mg sodium

---

Eat this: *Seafood linguine* 440 calories/1840 kJ, 19 g fat, 680 mg sodium

Not that: *Lasagne* 764 calories/3200 kJ, 43 g fat, 1360 mg sodium

---

Eat this: *Lemon sorbet (2 scoops)* 160 calories/672 kJ, 0 g fat, 18 mg sodium

Not that: *Tiramisu* 500 calories/2100 kJ, 20 g fat, 126 mg sodium

---

Chinese Restaurants

ABS DIET ENDORSEMENTS:

Chicken noodle soup 57 calories/237 kJ, 1 g fat, 900 mg sodium

Steamed dim sum (each) 69 calories/290 kJ, 4 g fat, 97 mg sodium

Steamed fish with ginger and spring onions 191 calories/805 kJ, 2 g fat, 965 mg sodium

Szechuan prawns with vegetables 332 calories/1388 kJ, 19 g fat, 2144 mg sodium

THE LESSER OF TWO EVILS

Eat this: *Spring roll (2 pieces)* 242 calories/1009 kJ, 16 g fat, 485 mg sodium	**Not that:** *Sesame prawn toasts* 402 calories/1689 kJ, 45 g fat, 865 mg sodium
Eat this: *Chicken and cashew nuts* 356 calories/1495 kJ, 16 g fat, 900 mg sodium	**Not that:** *Crispy duck* 497 calories/2063 kJ, 36 g fat, 680 mg sodium
Eat this: *Beef in black bean sauce* 448 calories/1881 kJ, 17 g fat, 600 mg sodium	**Not that:** *Sweet and sour pork (non battered)* 558 calories/2223 kJ, 26 g fat, 1482 mg sodium
Eat this: *Steamed rice* 414 calories/1761 kJ, 4 g fat, 4 mg sodium	**Not that:** *Egg fried rice* 558 calories/2361 kJ, 15 g fat, 1251 mg sodium
Eat this: *Lychees* 82 calories/348 kJ, 0 g fat, 2 mg sodium	**Not that:** *Toffee banana fritters* 370 calories/1554 kJ, 17 g fat, 810 mg sodium

Fish Restaurants

ABS DIET ENDORSEMENTS:

Grilled king prawns 164 calories/688 kJ, 3 g fat, 2440 mg sodium

Grilled plaice 200 calories/840 kJ, 4 g fat, 260 mg sodium

Grilled salmon steak 366 calories/1523 kJ, 22 g fat, 92 mg sodium

Salad with low-fat dressing 90 calories/378 kJ, 7 g fat, 490 mg sodium

THE LESSER OF TWO EVILS

Eat this: *Stuffed salmon* 495 calories/2058 kJ, 29 g fat, 346 mg sodium	**Not that:** *Battered cod* 556 calories/2320 kJ, 35 g fat, 360 mg sodium
Eat this: *New potatoes* 131 calories/562 kJ, 0.5 g fat, 16 mg sodium	**Not that:** *Chips* 502 calories/2102 kJ, 18 g fat, 74 mg sodium
Eat this: *Grilled whole lobster (without sauce)* 420 calories/1790 kJ, 12 g fat, 1200 mg sodium	**Not that:** *Spicy crab cakes with mayonnaise dip* 782 calories/3244 kJ, 65 g fat, 1245 mg sodium

Indian Restaurants

ABS DIET ENDORSEMENT:

Papadums (each) 65 calories/271 kJ, 5 g fat, 190 mg sodium

Chicken tikka 296 calories/1242 kJ, 11 g fat, 162 mg sodium

Sag bhaji 200 calories/830 kJ, 14 g fat, 1460 mg sodium

THE LESSER OF TWO EVILS

Eat this: *Plain boiled rice* 248 calories/1057 kJ, 2 g fat, 2 mg sodium	**Not that:** *Pilau rice* 256 calories/1078 kJ, 8 g fat, 198 mg sodium

Eat this: *Onion bhaji* 282 calories/1170 kJ, 18 g fat, 73 mg sodium	**Not that:** *Meat samosa* 381 calories/1590 kJ, 24 g fat, 573 mg sodium
Eat this: *Vegetable curry with rice* 563 calories/2371 kJ, 25 g fat, 1112 mg sodium	**Not that:** *Lamb biriani* 1104 calories/4616 kJ, 68 g fat, 1080 mg sodium
Eat this: *Chicken tikka masala* 471 calories/1968 kJ, 35 g fat, 1272 mg sodium	**Not that:** *Lamb kheema* 528 calories/2220 kJ, 40 g fat, 705 mg sodium

Thai Restaurants

ABS DIET ENDORSEMENT:

Tom yam (hot and sour prawn soup) 57 calories/237 kJ, 1 g fat, 900 mg sodium

Fish with ginger, garlic and chilli 197 calories/827 kJ, 2 g fat, 965 mg sodium

Gai pad krapow (stir-fried chicken with basil) 344 calories/1445 kJ, 8 g fat, 2189 mg sodium

THE LESSER OF TWO EVILS

Eat this: *Chicken satay* 287 calories/1197 kJ, 15 g fat, 920 mg sodium	**Not that:** *Thai fish cakes with peanut & chilli dip* 782 calories/3244 kJ, 65 g fat, 1245 mg sodium
Eat this: *Green chicken curry* 345 calories/1458 kJ, 8 g fat, 2300 mg sodium	**Not that:** *Lamb massaman curry* 1194 calories/4953 kJ, 100 g fat, 253 mg sodium
Eat this: *Stir-fried chicken with basil* 344 calories/1445 kJ, 8 g fat, 2189 mg sodium	**Not that:** *Pad thai (stir-fried rice noodles with beansprouts and peanuts)* 628 calories/2631 kJ, 31 g fat, 4268 mg sodium

Eat this: *Steamed jasmine rice* 414 calories/1761 kJ, 4 g fat, 3 mg sodium

Not that: *Coconut rice* 590 calories/2478 kJ, 15 g fat, 1251 mg sodium

---

Eat this: *Fresh mango* 86 calories/368 kJ, 0 g fat, 3 mg sodium

Not that: *Coconut ice cream* 258 calories/1073 kJ, 18 g fat, 72 mg sodium

---

Mexican Restaurants

ABS DIET ENDORSEMENTS:

Tortillas (each) 235 calories/979 kJ, 5 g fat, 344 mg sodium

Refried beans 237 calories/988 kJ, 3 g fat, 753 mg sodium

Salsa 40 calories/170 kJ, 0.2 g fat, 200 mg sodium

Chicken fajitas (each) 387 calories/1623 kJ, 10 g fat, 1050 mg sodium

THE LESSER OF TWO EVILS

Eat this: *Nachos with salsa and sour cream* 352 calories/1471 kJ, 21 g fat, 451 mg sodium

Not that: *Nachos with chicken and cheese* 606 calories/2528 kJ, 40 g fat, 804 mg sodium

---

Eat this: *Beef burrito* 662 calories/2768 kJ, 27 g fat, 1982 mg sodium

Not that: *Beef chimichanga (deep fried)* 850 calories/3554 kJ, 39 g fat, 1820 mg sodium

---

Eat this: *Chilli with rice* 542 calories/2283 kJ, 19 g fat, 669 mg sodium

Not that: *Beef enchilada* 646 calories/2700 kJ, 35 g fat, 2639 mg sodium

---

Eat this: *Refried beans* 237 calories/988 kJ, 3 g fat, 753 mg sodium

Not that: *Coleslaw* 387 calories/1409 kJ, 40 g fat, 240 mg sodium

Greek & Turkish Restaurants
ABS DIET ENDORSEMENTS:

Greek salad (side dish) 60 calories/252 kJ, 5 g fat, 330 mg sodium

Tzatziki 66 calories/275 kJ, 5 g fat, 372 mg sodium

Dolmades / stuffed vine leaves (each) 73 calories/307 kJ, 5 g fat, 287 mg sodium

Baked fish in vine leaves with oregano and tomato 280 calories/1172 kJ, 12 g fat, 795 mg sodium

THE LESSER OF TWO EVILS

Eat this: *Greek salad* 60 calories/252 kJ, 5 g fat, 330 mg sodium	**Not that:** *Deep-fried calamari and dip* 384 calories/1600 kJ, 24 g fat, 506 mg sodium
Eat this: *Baked feta cheese* 150 calories/622 kJ, 12 g fat, 864 mg sodium	**Not that:** *Taramasalata* 227 calories/935 kJ, 24 g fat, 293 mg sodium
Eat this: *Lamb souvlaki (kebabs)* 412 calories/1726 kJ, 20 g fat, 1020 mg sodium	**Not that:** *Moussaka* 607 calories/2354 kJ, 45 g fat, 1056 mg sodium
Eat this: *Greek yogurt with honey* 281 calories/1180 kJ, 13 g fat, 87 mg sodium	**Not that:** *Baklava (1 piece)* 322 calories/1349 kJ, 17 g fat, 310 mg sodium

Moroccan Restaurants
ABS DIET ENDORSEMENTS:

Harira soup (lentil) 218 calories/920 kJ, 8 g fat, 99 mg sodium

Hummus 112 calories/469 kJ, 7.6 g fat, 402 mg sodium

THE LESSER OF TWO EVILS

Eat this: *Mechoui (barbecued lamb)* 576 calories/2398 kJ, 39 g fat, 348 mg sodium	**Not that:** *Beef kofta* 706 calories/2938 kJ, 55 g fat, 1980 mg sodium
Eat this: *Vegetable couscous* 177 calories/748 kJ, 4 g fat, 100 mg sodium	**Not that:** *Lamb tagine* 415 calories/1751 kJ, 15 g fat, 313 mg sodium

Japanese Restaurants
ABS DIET ENDORSEMENTS:

Miso soup 39 calories/164 kJ, 3 g fat, 969 mg sodium

Sushi: Norimaki – seaweed-wrapped, with cucumber (each) 28 calories/117 kJ, 0.1 g fat, 208 mg sodium

Sushi: Nigiri – prawn (each) 36 calories/151 kJ, 0.1 g fat, 105 mg sodium

Sushi: Futomaki – crab and omelette (each) 73 calories/307 kJ, 1 g fat, 228 mg sodium

THE LESSER OF TWO EVILS

Eat this: *Mixed sushi* 270 calories/1134 kJ, 4 g fat, 612 mg sodium	**Not that:** *Prawn tempura (5 pieces)* 500 calories/2310 kJ, 35 g fat, 190 mg sodium
Eat this: *Noodle soup (large bowl)* 189 calories/792 kJ, 9 g fat, 420 mg sodium	**Not that:** *Katsu (breaded fried chicken)* 550 calories/2100 kJ, 15 g fat, 254 mg sodium

Eat this: *Salmon teriyaki* 363 calories/1514 kJ, 16 g fat, 2161 mg sodium

Not that: *Japanese pork curry* 457 calories/1924 kJ, 16 g fat, 1604 mg sodium

Pizza Places

Domino's Pizza

ABS DIET ENDORSEMENT:

Cheese & Tomato Deluxe Pizza (2 slices) 252 calories/1062 kJ, 6 g fat, 500 mg sodium

Veg-a-Roma Pizza (2 slices) 278 calories/1190 kJ, 8 g fat, 720 mg sodium

THE LESSER OF TWO EVILS

Eat this: *Hawaiian Pizza (2 slices)* 296 calories/1222 kJ, 6 g fat, 410 mg sodium

Not that: *Pepperoni Passion (2 slices)* 374 calories/1564 kJ, 15 g fat, 960 mg sodium

Eat this: *Garlic Pizza Bread (2 slices)* 224 calories/960 kJ, 7 g fat, 340 mg sodium

Not that: *Potato Wedges* 427 calories/1793 kJ, 17 g fat, 594 mg sodium

Eat this: *Chicken Strippers* 219 calories/920 kJ, 8 g fat, 400 mg sodium

Not that: *Chicken Combo* 552 calories/2315 kJ, 25 g fat, 1210 mg sodium

Eat this: *Cassis Royale* 290 calories/1217 kJ, 13 g fat, 66 mg sodium

Not that: *Hanky Panky Pie* 488 calories/2032 kJ, 31 g fat, 118 mg sodium

Pizza Hut

ABS DIET ENDORSEMENTS:

Salad Bowl (no extra dressings) 178 calories/677 kJ, 14 g fat, 98 mg sodium

THE LESSER OF TWO EVILS

Eat this: *Garlic Bread (4 slice portion)* 407 calories/1709 kJ, 16 g fat, 692 mg sodium	**Not that:** *Garlic Bread with Cheese (4 slice portion)* 587 calories/2457 kJ, 32 g fat, 1064 mg sodium
Eat this: *Mediterranean Vegetable Penne* 592 calories/2488 kJ, 20 g fat, 1204 mg sodium	**Not that:** *Tagliatelle Carbonara* 908 calories/3821 kJ, 52 g fat, 1744 mg sodium
Eat this: *Chicken Supreme individual pan pizza* 736 calories/3091 kJ, 30 g fat, 1600 mg sodium	**Not that:** *Chicken Feast individual pan pizza* 809 calories/3394 kJ, 34 g fat, 1600 mg sodium
Eat this: *Farmhouse individual pan pizza* 680 calories/2865 kJ 23 g fat, 1640 mg sodium	**Not that:** *Meat Feast individual pan pizza* 933 calories/3908 kJ, 47 g fat, 2240 mg sodium

DANGER AT YOUR DOORSTEP

The TV ads are tempting, but which delivery pizza will turn your Blockbuster night into your very own *Return of the Blob*?

Domino's *Cheese & Tomato Deluxe Pizza (2 slices)* 252 calories/1062 kJ, 6 g fat, 500 mg sodium

Pizza Hut *Margherita individual pan pizza* 809 calories/3401 kJ, 34 g fat, 1360 mg sodium

Papa John's *The Classic Pizza (1 slice 35 cm/14 in pizza)* 295 calories/1239 kJ, 10 g fat, 702 mg sodium

Papa John's/Perfect Pizza

ABS DIET ENDORSEMENTS:

The Classic Pizza (1 slice 35 cm / 14 in pizza) 295 calories/1239 kJ, 10 g fat, 702 mg sodium

Breadsticks (per stick) 140 calories/588 kJ, 2 g fat, 260 mg sodium

Pizza Dipping Sauce 20 calories/84 kJ, 0 g fat, 310 mg sodium

THE LESSER OF TWO EVILS

Eat this: *Hawaiian Pizza (1 slice 35 cm/14 in pizza)* 296 calories/1243 kJ, 9 g fat, 806 mg sodium	**Not that:** *Papa's Pepperoni Plus pizza (1 slice 35 cm/14 in pizza)* 342 calories/1436 kJ, 15 g fat, 912 mg sodium
Eat this: *Garden Special Pizza (1 slice 35 cm/14 in pizza)* 286 calories/1201 kJ, 9 g fat, 700 mg sodium	**Not that:** *The Works Pizza (1 slice 35 cm/14 in pizza)* 369 calories/1550 kJ,16 g fat, 1012 mg sodium
Eat this: *Breadsticks (2 pieces)* 280 calories/1176 kJ, 4 g fat, 520 mg sodium	**Not that:** *Garlic Cheesesticks (2 pieces)* 360 calories/1512 KJ, 16 g fat, 830 mg sodium
Eat this: *Papa's Chicken Dippers with Buffalo dipping sauce* 175 calories/735 kJ, 8.5 g fat, 1240 mg sodium	**Not that:** *Papa's Chicken Dippers with Garlic dipping sauce* 310 calories/1302 kJ, 24 g fat, 670 mg sodium

Smoothies

I prefer it if you make your own smoothie, but sometimes you need one on the go. If so, always get yours with extra protein (you'd be surprised how many of these shakes are just fruit, water and air). Make sure the shake contains a gram or two of fat, otherwise your body won't absorb many of the fat-soluble nutrients from all that fruit. Simply asking for it to be made with low-fat milk or yogurt will do the trick. But beware fat bombs. Here's a clue: if the dairy element doesn't state 'low-fat', it probably isn't.

Boost Juice

ABS DIET ENDORSEMENTS:

All Berry Bang (450ml) 311 calories/1300 kJ, 5 g fat, 58 mg sodium

Skinny Dip (450 ml) 333 calories/1390 kJ, 5 g fat, 59 mg sodium

THE LESSER OF TWO EVILS

Drink this: *Energy Lift (450 ml)* 333 calories/1390 kJ, 5 g fat, 58 mg sodium	**Not that:** *King William Chocolate (450 ml)* 404 calories/1690 kJ, 6 g fat, 248 mg sodium
Drink this: *Gym Junkie (450 ml)* 373 calories/1560 kJ, 5.5 g fat, 231 mg sodium	**Not that:** *Breakie to Go-Go (450 ml)* 572 calories/2390 kJ, 10 g fat, 288 mg sodium

Crussh

ABS DIET ENDORSEMENTS:

Super Juice (350 ml / 12 fl oz) 91 calories/385 kJ, 1.5 g fat, 2100 mg sodium

Berry Blast (350 ml / 12 fl oz) 287 calories/1205 kJ, 3.5 g fat, 0 mg sodium

Good Morning (350 ml / 12 fl oz) 295 calories/1240 kJ, 4 g fat, 0 mg sodium

THE LESSER OF TWO EVILS

Drink this: *Strawberry Cool (350 ml/12 fl oz)* 270 calories/1132 kJ, 3.5 g fat, 0 mg sodium	**Not that:** *Bananarama (350 ml/12 fl oz)* 342 calories/1437 kJ, 3.5 g fat, 350 mg sodium
Eat this: *Tangy Prawn Cocktail Sandwich* 342 calories/1436 kJ, 7 g fat, 1200 mg sodium	**Not that:** *Smokey Ham Swiss Sandwich* 495 calories/2073 kJ, 21 g fat, 530 mg sodium

Ice Cream Shops

Firstly, come here directly after a meal. You'll be less likely to pig out. Secondly, don't stress too much about it; ice cream may be sugary and high in calories, but it also provides protein and calcium. As indulgences go, it's hardly a high crime. So don't waste your time on nasty no-sugar-added ice creams; no sense eating food you don't enjoy. Instead, look for reduced-fat options and add Powerfoods (nuts and fruit) whenever possible. And if you completely ignore all that advice, take this tip: order the ice cream you absolutely love . . . in a single-scoop cup.

Baskin-Robbins

ABS DIET ENDORSEMENTS:

Low-fat Vanilla Ice Cream (3 scoops) 164 calories/690 kJ, 2.5 g fat, 125 mg sodium

Light Espresso & Cream Low-fat Ice Cream (3 scoops) 186 calories/784 kJ, 4.5 g fat, 120 mg sodium

Lemon Sorbet (3 scoops) 133 calories/557 kJ, 0 g fat, 15 mg sodium

Chocolate Chip No-sugar-added Ice Cream (3 scoops) 136 calories/575 kJ, 3.5 g fat, 150 mg sodium

THE LESSER OF TWO EVILS

Eat this: *Chocolate Ice Cream (3 scoops)* 263 calories/1106 kJ, 8 g fat, 125 mg sodium	**Not that:** *2-scoop Hot Chocolate Fudge Sundae* 530 calories/2226 kJ, 29 g fat, 200 mg sodium
Eat this: *Mango Tango Ice Cream (3 scoops)* 237 calories/997 kJ, 10 g fat, 85 mg sodium	**Not that:** *Caramel Chocolate Crunch (3 scoops)* 295 calories/1243 kJ, 15 g fat, 150 mg sodium

Häagen-Dazs

ABS DIET ENDORSEMENTS:

Zesty Lemon Sorbet (3 scoops) 110 calories/462 kJ, 0 g fat, 25 mg sodium

Chocolate Sorbet (3 scoops) 130 calories/546 kJ, 0 g fat, 70 mg sodium

Chocolate Fudge Brownie Frozen Yogurt (3 scoops) 200 calories/840 kJ, 2.5 g fat, 140 mg sodium

Vanilla Frozen Yogurt (3 scoops) 200 calories/840 kJ, 4.5 g fat, 55 mg sodium

THE LESSER OF TWO EVILS

Eat this: *Dulce de Leche Frozen Yogurt (3 scoops)* 190 calories/798 kJ, 2.5 g fat, 75 mg sodium

Not that: *Butter Pecan Ice Cream (3 scoops)* 310 calories/1302 kJ, 23 g fat, 100 mg sodium

Eat this: *Pineapple Coconut Ice Cream (3 scoops)* 230 calories/966 kJ, 13 g fat, 55 mg sodium

Not that: *Chocolate Chip Cookie Dough Ice Cream (3 scoops)* 310 calories/1302 kJ, 20 g fat, 125 mg sodium

HE WANTED TO CHASE AFTER HIS KIDS, SO HE CHASED AFTER A GOAL

Name: William Salerno

Age: 38

Height: 1.75 m/5'9"

Weight, Week 1: 100 kg/15 st 12 lb

Weight, Week 6: 90 kg/14 st 2 lb

Having twins 2 years ago meant that William Salerno was going to be busier than ever. He was in a job that routinely required him to work 12-hour days, plus now he had to help care for two young children. And that's when it hit him.

'I feel like I'm an older dad and that I gotta stay ahead of these guys,' Salerno says. 'I want to be like my father was with me – always active. And that got me thinking.'

That's when his business manager told him he had to read *The Abs Diet*.

'When I read it, something clicked. I'm amazed by it because I usually don't go for those kinds of books. Usually they don't do anything for me,' he says. 'I started to read it in my office one day and read it for a couple hours. I carried it everywhere. Now I talk about trans fats and high-fructose corn syrup to anybody who'll listen to me.'

He reads food ingredients on everything – and remains pumped up about the plan.

'Almonds are a godsend,' he says.

A side benefit is that he no longer experiences any symptoms with gout – a disorder that causes pain in the joints that's hampered Salerno in the past.

'My theory is that if I'm 100 kg/15 st 12 lb, then I could very well have been 105 kg/16 st 6 lb – I was in that range for a couple of years,' Salerno says. 'People see me now and they say, where'd it all go? They think I'm starving myself, and I'm not. It's so refreshing and unbelievable.'

Now, he can't stop talking about it.

'I quoted passages to my wife so often that she began calling me "the *Abs Diet* zealot".'

Chapter 10

INDULGE AND ENJOY

The Abs Diet Seasonal Survival Guide

IF A DIET IS AN ANT, then the holiday season is the bottom of a shoe, because it has the power to squash you every time. Between the mince pies, sausages, more mince pies, drinks, fruitcake, roast potatoes and gravy (oh, the gravy), many of us cram 6 months of eating into 6 weeks. The result: come January, the only thing you're trying to cram is extra flab into your jeans.

As you know, the Abs Diet isn't about deprivation, so I want you to have the occasional tussle with a kilo-high mound of stuffing. If you do that for 6 weeks straight, you'll have succeeded – on the Flabs Diet. Since you have one cheat meal per week, I suggest you play your card around the biggest bomb – whether it's Christmas dinner, the New Year's Eve party or a date with Aunt Matilda's can't-resist chocolate cheesecake – and then sidestep the dietary land mines through the rest of the week. To eat right throughout the holidays, these choices will help you avoid turning your diet into a disaster.

Christmas Dinner

THE LESSER OF TWO EVILS

Eat this: *225 g/8 oz roast turkey breast*	**Not that:** *225 g/8 oz roast turkey dark meat*
4 roast potatoes	*6 roast potatoes*
4 roast parsnips	*6 roast parsnips*
100 g/3½ oz brussels sprouts	*100 g/3½ oz stuffing*
4 tablespoons turkey gravy	*8 tablespoons turkey gravy*
1 tablespoon cranberry sauce	*2 tablespoons cranberry sauce*
1 sliver Christmas pudding	*1 portion Christmas pudding*
2 teaspoons brandy butter	*2 teaspoons brandy butter*
TOTAL: 1242 calories/5216 kJ, 43 g fat (13 g saturated), 787 mg sodium	TOTAL: 2090 calories/8795 kJ, 87 g fat (25 g saturated), 1675 mg sodium

Christmas Leftovers

THE LESSER OF TWO EVILS

Eat this: *115 g/4 oz turkey breast on 2 pieces wholegrain bread with mustard and lettuce* 352 calories/1478 kJ, 4.5 g fat (1 g saturated), 432 mg sodium	**Not that:** *115 g/4 oz turkey on soft white roll with butter and mayo* 598 calories/2497 kJ, 38 g fat (11 g saturated), 565 mg sodium
Eat this: *Mince pie* 239 calories/1004 kJ, 12 g fat (4 g saturated), 156 mg sodium	**Not that:** *Christmas cake* 350 calories/1478 kJ, 10 g fat (2 g saturated), 113 mg sodium
Eat this: *Fruit salad (with juice. not syrup)* 118 calories/462 kJ, 0.2 g fat, 5 mg sodium	**Not that:** *Sherry trifle* 282 calories/1178 kJ, 16 g fat (9 g saturated), 107 mg sodium

New Year's Eve Party

THE LESSER OF TWO EVILS

Drink this: *Champagne* 90 calories/377 kJ, 0 g fat, 0 mg sodium

Not that: *Vodka and tonic* 125 calories/523 kJ, 0 g fat, 7 mg sodium

---

Eat this: *12 large prawns with 2 tablespoons cocktail sauce* 192 calories/802 kJ, 10 g fat (0.2 g saturated), 1796 mg sodium

Not that: *4 cocktail sausages* 328 calories/1377 kJ, 27 g fat (10 g saturated), 807 mg sodium

---

Eat this: *8 melon balls wrapped in prosciutto* 220 calories/924 kJ, 11 g fat (4 g saturated), 1650 mg sodium

Not that: *3 blinis with sour cream, smoked salmon and caviar* 290 calories/1214 kJ, 12 g fat (4 g saturated), 1760 mg sodium

---

Eat this: *Sliced raw vegetables (unlimited) with 50 g guacamole* 110 calories/452 kJ, 10 g fat (3 g saturated), 285 mg sodium

Not that: *50 g potato crisps (chips)* 265 calories/1110 kJ, 17 g fat (7 g saturated), 400 mg sodium

---

Eat this: *60 g/2 oz Camembert and 20 grapes* 198 calories/826 kJ, 14 g fat (6 g saturated), 364 mg sodium

Not that: *2 small slices quiche* 300 calories/1256 kJ, 22 g fat (9 g saturated), 348 mg sodium

---

Feasts, Not Famine

At the end of the year, you're tempted everywhere – at meals, by the office chocolates, under the mistletoe. If you can make it through the biggest fat wave of the year, the other 11 months will be smoother than a supermodel's freshly shaved legs. Sure, you'll hit the occasional feast. Go ahead and enjoy them, but know that you can always make decisions to satisfy your tastes and cravings without drowning yourself in fat.

Easter Dinner

THE LESSER OF TWO EVILS

Eat this: *225 g/8 oz roast lamb* *4 roast potatoes with olive oil* *100 g/3½ oz steamed spinach* TOTAL: 774 calories/3258 kJ, 31 g fat (9 g saturated), 280 mg sodium

Not that: *225 g/8 oz roast ham* *creamy mashed potatoes* *200 g/7 oz broad beans in parsley sauce* TOTAL: 858 calories/3598 kJ, 40 g fat (15 g saturated), 2898 mg sodium

Eat this: *1 hot cross bun, no butter* 156 calories/660 kJ, 3 g fat (1 g saturated), 47 mg sodium

Not that: *1 slice chocolate cake* 443 calories/1854 kJ, 24 g fat (13 g saturated), 260 mg sodium

World Cup Party

THE LESSER OF TWO EVILS

Eat this: *2 handfuls unsalted nuts*
Baked tortilla chips with salsa
2 slices chicken or turkey breast or
lean roast beef
Wholemeal roll
TOTAL: 720 calories/3019 kJ,
37 g fat (7 g saturated), 715 mg
sodium

Not that: *Celery with onion dip*
Nachos with cheese dip
15 chicken wings
TOTAL: 1264 calories/5308 kJ,
86 g fat (26 g saturated), 2229 mg
sodium

Barbecues

THE LESSER OF TWO EVILS

Eat this: *1 quarter-pound grilled*
burger with ketchup, mustard,
lettuce, tomato, slice of cheese
115 g/4 oz homemade coleslaw
TOTAL: 426 calories/1776 kJ, 30 g
fat (14 g saturated), 1062 mg
sodium

Not that: *2 sausages*
115 g/4 oz potato salad
TOTAL: 565 calories/2199 kJ,
48 g fat (11 g saturated), 1048 mg
sodium

Eat this: *Fish, shellfish and pep-*
per (capsicum) kebab 208 calo-
ries/872 kJ, 7 g fat (1 g saturated),
853 mg sodium

Not that: *2 chicken legs* 780 calo-
ries/3276 kJ, 56 g fat (15 g saturated), 314 mg sodium

Eat this: *Medium baked potato*
with butter 319 calories/1352 kJ,
9 g fat (5 g saturated), 82 mg
sodium

Not that: *French fries* 420 calo-
ries/1764 kJ, 16 g fat (9 g saturated), 465 mg sodium

Sweets and Treats
THE LESSER OF TWO EVILS

Eat this: *Kit Kat (2-finger bar)* 106 calories/444 kJ, 5 g fat (3 g saturated), 12 mg sodium

Not that: *Chocolate-coated honeycomb crunch bar* 210 calories/880 kJ, 8 g fat (6 g saturated), 90 mg sodium

Eat this: *Milky Way (fun-size bar):* 76 calories/318 kJ, 3 g fat (1 g saturated), 43 mg sodium

Not that: *Mars Bar (fun-size bar):* 100 calories /418 kJ, 4 g fat (2 g saturated), 45 mg sodium

Eat this: *Jelly beans (about 20 pieces)* 82 calories/343 kJ, 0 g fat, 11 mg sodium

Not that: *Werther's Original (6 pieces):* 130 calories/544kJ, 3 g fat (2 g saturated), 120 mg sodium

Eat this: *3 After Eight Mints* 90 calories/377 kJ, 3 g fat (2 g saturated), 3 mg sodium

Not that: *1 Cadbury's Creme Egg* 170 calories/712 kJ, 6 g fat (3.5 g saturated), 25 mg sodium

Eat this: *1 handful roasted pistachios* 175 calories/752 kJ, 14 g fat (1.7 g saturated), 125 mg sodium

Not that: *1 handful M&M's* 256 calories/1072 kJ, 11 g fat (7 g saturated), 32 mg sodium

Eat this: *1 brownie (5 cm/2 in square)* 165 calories/690 kJ, 7 g fat (2 g saturated), 82 mg sodium

Not that: *A few chunks of peanut brittle* 274 calories/1147 kJ, 11 g fat (2 g saturated), 252 mg sodium

Chapter 11

CRANK UP THE FAT BURN

The Abs Diet Workout

BETWEEN YOUR JOB, family, home, and Google addiction, you probably feel pushed and pulled in more directions than a piece of Play Doh. Me, too.

The clock seems to move faster and faster, and we're all running to keep up. We crave less stress, more time, and 30 uninterrupted seconds during which nobody nags us about meeting deadlines, caulking cracks, or playing a 14th consecutive game of Cluedo.

We're all busy. But we're not too busy to exercise.

Here's the proof: the average person spends 28 hours a week watching television. If you watch only half as much TV, that still means you have more than a full working day of quality time you're spending in the Big Brother house, on Ramsay Street, or on the sofa with Richard and Judy every week.

Give up just one of those hours each week – just one – and you can change your body and your life for ever.

I said at the very beginning of this book that the Abs Diet was no ordinary diet, and I meant it. To me, one of the biggest errors in most mainstream diets is that they treat exercise the way the prom queen treats the chess champ – with indifference. They operate on ho-hum exercise principles: great if you do it, so what if you don't.

But most plans overlook one simple truth: the best way to lose fat is to build muscle and let that muscle eat away flab from the inside out. Each 455 g/1 lb of muscle you build means your body will burn up to an extra 50 calories a day just sitting still. Add 2.25 kg/5 lb of muscle – something you can easily do over the course of 6 weeks – and you're now burning up to an extra 1,750 calories a week! When it comes down to it, exercise can do just as much to reshape your body as any broccoli floret can.

Of course, the ABS DIET POWER 12 gives you all the weapons you need to fight fat: protein, healthy fat, whole grains and fibre to keep you full, to feed your body nutrients and to ward off potentially devastating hunger pangs. But you'll accelerate all of your gains with the secret weapon in your dietary artillery: muscle.

I'm not talking bar-bouncer, piano-lifting muscle. I'm talking about lean muscle mass, which works as your body's natural metabolism booster. To make the Abs Diet as effective as possible, you need to add a muscle-building and strength-training workout to your programme.

Now, if the only dumbbells you know live four doors down, then the prospect of taking up strength training may seem intimidating. It shouldn't be. Like the Abs Diet itself, the Abs Diet Workout is designed to be fast, simple, effective and convenient. I know you're not going to spend hours a day in the gym, I know you're not going to enjoy a workout programme that's all pain and no gain, and I know you're not going to stick with it if you don't see impressive results, fast. That's why I've created a workout programme that will build muscle, melt away fat and reintroduce you to your abs – all in just 20 minutes a day, 3 days a week.

How do I know it works? Besides the countless success stories of people who reshaped their bodies with minimal time at the gym, one study found that you can put on 2.75 kg/6 lb of muscle and lose 6.8 kg/15 lb of fat in 6 weeks by following the exercise principles used in the Abs Diet Workout. We're talking just 20 minutes a day, just 3 days a week.

Don't believe it? Think you need to quit your job and spend your life in the gym to see results? Well, check this out: scientists at the University of Glamorgan in Wales studied 16 weightlifters doing either one or three sets of upper-body exercises three times a week. Those who did one set gained just as much muscle – and burned twice as much fat – as the three-set group. In other words, the less time you spend, the better your results!

What's great about this programme is that you can do it in a gym or in your house, you don't need fancy equipment, and you can finish it before *ER* is even halfway over. (In fact, I've even included a no-weight workout that you can do in your garden, in a hotel room, in a prison cell if need be. No excuses, remember?) One hour a week. That's all I want, and that's all you need.

Your 3-Days-a-Week Muscle-Building, Fat-Burning Programme

Think of muscle as your body's python and fat as a quivering mouse. In the battle between the two, the python will always win. And the bigger your python, the more mice it eats.

What's great about weight training is that it burns fat in three ways. Firstly, there are the calories you burn off breaking a sweat. Secondly, there's the fact that new muscle eats up calories, making your body more efficient at burning fat. And thirdly, there's the 'afterburn' – the additional calories burned off in the hours immediately following your workout. All kinds of exercise raise your metabolism and give you an afterburn. But the effects of weight training far outstrip those of aerobic exercise. In one study, researchers found that the increased calorie burn of aerobics (that is, steady-state cardiovascular exercise like running or cycling) lasted only 30 minutes to an hour after a workout. In subjects who trained with weights, the increased metabolism lasted as long as 48 hours. That's 2 days during which your body burns fat after the fact.

And you don't need to push iron like Arnie to achieve the afterburn effect. All you have to do is employ the two major Abs Diet components of muscle building: circuit training and compound exercises.

Circuit training. There are many different ways to lift weights. A lot of people employ the lift-rest-lift-rest approach to weight training, and that's fine. But my guess is that you're interested in building the most muscle and burning the most fat in the least amount of time possible. So I've built the Abs Diet Workout around circuit training. In this type of training, there is no rest phase, no part of the workout where you're standing around the water fountain looking lost. Circuit training means that your body is constantly working, constantly improving.

BONUS: ADVANCED ABS!

If you're starting to feel as if your abs are tighter than the jeans you just pulled out of the dryer, then you're probably ready for a more challenging abdominal exercise. Try this one. Lie on your back on a Swiss ball, with your knees bent at 90 degrees, your feet flat and your hands behind your ears. Keeping your right foot planted, lift your left foot off the floor and bring it towards you as you curl your torso up and to the left so that your right elbow meets your left knee. It's like the classic bicycle manoeuvre, and it works your entire core at once. Do 12 repetitions. Then plant your left foot on the floor and curl towards your right knee for another 12 reps.

Simply put, circuit training involves moving from one exercise to the next with little rest in between. Once you complete the circuit of 9 or 11 exercises, you rest for 2 minutes and then start again. In your time-compressed life, circuit training works because it means you're working the most muscles in the least amount of time; plus, with little rest, your heart rate stays elevated to give you an additional calorie burn. A recent Ohio University study found that a short-but-hard workout was effective in burning fat. Using a circuit of three exercises in a row for 31 minutes, the subjects were still burning more calories than normal 38 hours after the workout.

Compound exercises. Just like compound interest, compound exercises give you more back than you put in. Compound exercises hit many muscles during a single move (the squat engages 256 muscles at once!), so that you're gaining the most benefit from your workout. Compound exercises also ensure that you work the largest muscles in your body (like your chest, legs and back). Larger muscles take more calories to maintain than smaller ones, making your workout that much more effective.

To put it all together, all you need is a gym membership or, if you're exercising at home, a set of dumbbells and a bench. (For dumbbells, I recommend you invest in an adjustable pair so that you can change weights for different exercises and up the resistance as you grow stronger.) Though it doesn't matter where you do the circuit, it does matter when you do it. Stick to 3 days a week with at least 1 day a week of rest in between to allow your muscles to recover and grow.

The Abs Diet Circuit

Perform each exercise once, then move immediately to the next exercise with only 30 seconds of rest in between. When you reach the end of the circuit, rest for 2 minutes and then repeat.

Beginners can start with light weights and one circuit. More advanced lifters can do two or three circuits with weights that they can comfortably handle for at least 8 repetitions but no more than 12 repetitions.

ULTIMATE NO-WEIGHT WORKOUT

Sometimes, you can't get to the gym or even access the workout gear you have stashed in your cellar. Maybe you're stuck in some godforsaken motel. Maybe you're trapped at your in-laws' house. Maybe you're helping the police with their enquiries. Well, that's still no excuse. This full-body routine requires no equipment and only 8 minutes of your time. Perform each exercise below for 30 seconds. Do one move after another without rest and repeat the sequence without rest for a total of four times, if you can.

The intensity of this workout conditions your muscular and cardiovascular systems, helps improve flexibility and melts fat. You'll burn hundreds of calories.

Jumping Jack. Just like primary school. Start with your hands on your hips and your feet together. Raise your hands out to your sides and up overhead as you move your feet out to the sides. Then bring your feet back together and lower your hands to your sides.

Split Hop. Stand with your hands on your hips and your feet together. Move your left foot 15 cm/6 in forward and your right foot 15 cm/6 in back. Now jump up and switch legs so that your right foot is forward.

Squat Thrust with Press-up. Stand with your arms at your sides. Bend your knees and lower your hands to the floor. Kick your legs behind you so that you're in a press-up position. Now do a press-up. Thrust your knees to your chest so that your feet are back underneath you and stand back up.

Mountain Climber. Get back in the press-up position and kick your knees to your chest, one leg at a time. Alternate thrusting your knees forward, like you're running, so that one leg is extended when one knee is forward.

EXERCISE	REPETITIONS	REST	SETS
Squat	10–12	30 seconds	2
Bench Press	10	30 seconds	2
Pulldown	10	30 seconds	2
Military Press	10	30 seconds	2
Upright Row	10	30 seconds	2
Triceps Pushdown	10–12	30 seconds	2
Leg Extension	10–12	30 seconds	2
Biceps Curl	10	30 seconds	2
Leg Curl	10–12	30 seconds	2

Note: One day a week, add the following two exercises (do the Travelling Lunge after the Pulldown, and the Step-Up after the Upright Row). Because your legs contain your body's largest muscles, the fat-burning potential increases with a little extra time spent working your legs muscles.

EXERCISE	REPETITIONS	REST	SETS
Travelling Lunge	10–12 (each leg)	30 seconds	2
Step-Up	10–12 (each leg)	30 seconds	2

Squat. Hold a barbell with an overhand grip so that it rests comfortably on your upper back. Set your feet shoulder-width apart, and keep your knees slightly bent, back straight and eyes focused straight ahead. Slowly lower your body as if you were sitting back into a chair, keeping your back in its natural alignment and your lower legs perpendicular to the floor. When your thighs are parallel to the floor, pause, then return to the starting position.

Home variation: Same, but with one dumbbell in each hand, your palms facing your outer thighs.

Bench Press. Lie on your back on a flat bench with your feet on the floor. Grab the barbell with an overhand grip, your hands just beyond shoulder-width apart. Lift the bar off the uprights and hold it at arm's length over your chest. Slowly lower the bar to your chest. Pause, then push the bar back to the starting position.

Home variation: Press-ups. Get in a press-up position with your hands shoulder-width apart. Bend at the elbows while keeping your back straight, until your chin almost touches the floor, then push back up.

Pulldown. Stand facing a lat pulldown machine. Reach up and grasp the bar with an overhand grip that's 10 to 15 cm/4 to 6 in wider than your shoulders. Sit on the seat, letting the resistance of the bar extend your arms above your head. When you're in position, pull the bar down until it touches your upper chest. Hold the position for a second, then return to the starting position.

Home variation: Bent-Over Row. Stand with your knees slightly bent and shoulder-width apart. Bend over so that your back is almost parallel to the floor. Holding a dumbbell in each hand, let your arms hang towards the floor. With your palms facing in, pull the dumbbells towards you until they touch the outside of your chest. Pause, then return to the starting position.

Military Press. Sitting on an exercise bench, hold a barbell at shoulder height with your hands shoulder-width apart. Press the weight straight overhead so that your arms are almost fully extended, hold for a count of one, then bring it down to the front of your shoulders.

Home variation: Sitting on a sturdy chair instead of a bench, hold one dumbbell in each hand, about level with your ears. Push the dumbbells straight overhead so that your arms are almost fully extended, hold for a count of one, then return to the starting position.

Upright Row. Grab a barbell with an overhand grip and stand with your feet shoulder-width apart and your knees slightly bent. Let the barbell hang at arm's length on top of your thighs, thumbs pointed towards each other. Bending your elbows, lift your upper arms straight out to the sides and pull the barbell straight up until your upper arms are parallel to the floor and the bar is just below chin level. Pause, then return to the starting position.

Home variation: Same, using one dumbbell in each hand.

Triceps Pushdown. While standing, grip a bar attached to a high pulley cable or lat machine with your hands 15 cm/6 in apart. With your elbows tucked against your sides, bring the bar down until it is directly in front of you. With your forearms parallel to the floor (the starting position), push the bar down until your arms are extended straight down with the bar near your thigh. Don't lock your elbows. Return to the starting position.

Home variation: Triceps Kickback. Holding a light dumbbell in each hand, stand with your knees slightly bent and shoulder-width apart. Bend over so that your back is almost parallel to the ground. Bend your elbows to about 90-degree angles, raising them to just above the level of your back. This is the starting position. Extend your forearms backwards, keeping your upper arms stationary. When they're fully extended, your arms should be parallel to the ground. Pause, then return to the starting position.

WHAT'S MY MOTIVATION?

No matter how dedicated you are to your weight-loss goals, there are some days when you don't feel like getting out of bed, much less getting to the gym. How do you keep making progress? Here are a few tricks to keep you from falling off the exercise wagon.

Make a bet. Challenge a colleague to a contest – the first to lose 4.5 kg/10 lb, best of seven in one-on-one, and so forth. Competition is the ultimate motivator.

Switch training partners. Working out with a partner who will hold you accountable for showing up at the gym works well – for a while. But the longer you know him, the easier it is to back out of a workout. Find a new one every few months.

Strike an agreement with your family. The rule: you get 1 hour to yourself every day, provided that you use it for exercise (and reciprocate the favour).

Schedule a body-composition test every 2 months. The short-term end date will keep you focused to keep moving forward.

Leg Extension. Sitting on a leg extension machine with your feet under the footpads, lean back slightly and lift the pads with your feet until your legs are extended.

Home variation: Stand with your back flat against a wall. Squat down so that your thighs are parallel to the ground. Hold that position for as long as you can. That consists of one set. Aim for 20 seconds to start and work your way up to 45 seconds.

Biceps Curl. Stand while holding a barbell in front of you, palms facing out, with your hands shoulder-width apart and your arms hanging in front of you. Curl the weight towards your shoulders, hold for a second, then return to the starting position.

Home variation: Same, only use a set of dumbbells instead.

Leg Curl. Lie facedown on a leg curl machine and hook your ankles under the padded bar. Keeping your stomach and pelvis against the bench, slowly raise your feet towards your buttocks, curling up the weight. Come up so that your feet nearly touch your buttocks, and slowly return to the starting position.

Home variation: Lie down with your stomach on the floor. Put a light dumbbell between your feet (so that the top end of the dumbbell rests on the bottom of your feet). Squeeze your feet together and curl them up towards your buttocks.

Travelling Lunge. Rest a barbell against your upper back. Stand, with your feet hip-width apart, at one end of the room; you need room to walk about 20 steps. Step forward with your left foot, and lower your body so that your left thigh is parallel to the floor and your right thigh is perpendicular to the floor (your right knee should bend and almost touch the floor). Stand and bring your right foot up next to your left, then repeat with the right leg lunging forward.

Home variation: Use dumbbells, holding one in each hand with your arms at your sides. If you don't have enough space, do the move in one place, alternating your lead foot with each lunge.

Step-Up. Use a step or bench that's 45 cm/18 in off the ground. Place your left foot on the step so that your knee is bent at 90 degrees. Your knee should not advance past the toes of your left foot. Push off with your left foot and bring your right foot onto the step, keeping your back straight. Now step down with the left foot, followed by the right. Alternate the leading foot, or do all of the repetitions leading with one foot and then alternating. Once you're comfortable, add dumbbells.

Home variation: Same, only use a staircase instead of a step (if you don't have one).

Abdominal Exercises: Before Your Circuit

You'd think with a name like the Abs Diet, I'd be asking you to spend more time working your abs than J.Lo spends working the counters at Tiffany & Co. But finding your abs isn't as much about abdominal exercises as it is about changing your body composition to eliminate the fat that's covering them. Once you do that, then you can concentrate on building the muscle. It's sort of like a construction company trying to build a housing development. If you don't clear the site of sand, debris and trees, you aren't going to have any room to build the house. But if you clear the site and lay the foundation, then you can build a house that everyone will see.

To work your abs, you'll want to hit all five parts of your abdominal region (as outlined below). At the beginning of your strength circuit (2 or 3 days a week), do these five exercises in a circuit with little rest in between each. Start with one set, but work up to doing two or three sets. To vary your exercises, see *The Abs Diet*, which has 50 variations of abdominal moves.

Traditional Crunch (works the upper part of the rectus abdominis, which is the six-pack muscle that helps you maintain good posture). Lie on your back with your knees bent and your hands behind your ears. Slowly crunch up, bringing your shoulder blades off the ground. Do 12 to 15 repetitions.

Flutter Kick (works the lower part of the rectus abdominis). Lie on your back, raise both feet off the ground, and scissor-kick one leg over the other. Do 20 repetitions.

Saxon Side Bend (works the external and internal obliques, which extend diagonally down the sides of your waist and rotate the torso). Hold a pair of lightweight dumbbells over your head, in line with your shoulders, with your elbows slightly bent. Keep your back straight, and slowly bend directly to your left side as far as possible without twisting your upper body. Pause, return to an upright position, then bend to your right side as far as possible. Do 6 to 10 repetitions.

Bridge (works the transverse abdominis, which is known as the girdle because it compresses the abdomen). Start to get in a press-up position, but bend your elbows and rest your weight on your forearms instead. Your body should form a straight line. Pull your abdominals in. Hold for 20 seconds, breathing steadily. Do 1 to 2 repetitions.

Superman (works the lower back, which anchors all of the abdominal muscles). Lie with your stomach on the ground and your arms in front of you and legs behind you (in Superman-flying position). Lift your arms and legs about 15 cm/6 in off the ground and hold for as long as you can. Repeat three times.

Interval Training: 1 Day a Week

Back in the '80s, the only thing more popular than big hair and shoulder pads was running. Weight-loss experts touted long, steady aerobic exercise as nearly the best way to burn fat, build endurance and keep the heart pumping.

And aerobic exercise (running, cycling, swimming) is good for you. I've run the New York City Marathon twice myself, and I can attest to the fact that cardiovascular exercise strengthens your heart, burns calories and decreases stress.

But cardio has two significant drawbacks. Firstly, it only burns calories while you're doing it, not afterwards. Secondly, it does nothing to build muscle. Unless . . . unless you try interval training.

Interval training refers to a shorter, more intense method of working out. Instead of long, slow, boring runs or rides, interval training intersperses short bursts of high-intensity exertion with periods of slow, more restful exercise. In a Canadian study from Laval University, researchers measured differences in fat loss between two groups of exercisers following two different workout programmes. The first group rode stationary bikes at a steady pace four or five times a week and burned 300 to 400 calories per 30- to 45-minute session. The second group did the same, but only one or two times a week, and they filled the rest of their sessions with short intervals of high-intensity cycling. They hopped on

ULTIMATE TOTAL-BODY DUMBBELL EXERCISE

Dumbbells are one of the smartest fitness investments you can make. They're portable and affordable, and they condition your body even more effectively than standard barbells, because they teach your body to balance and allow for a greater range of motion.

I've created here a super-simple, super-fast dumbbell workout that will hit your whole body at once. Do one set of 12 repetitions, and you're set for the day.

▶ Grab a pair of light dumbbells and get into a press-up position, with your arms straight and directly beneath your shoulders.

▶ Do a press-up. Then bring your feet underneath you, one foot at a time.

▶ Keeping your back flat, stand up. (This is a deadlift.)

▶ From the standing position, curl the weights up to your shoulders.

▶ Swing your elbows out to your sides so that the weights are above your shoulders.

▶ Lower your body until your thighs are parallel to the floor. Pause, then stand up as you press the weights overhead.

their stationary bikes and pedalled as quickly as they could for 30 to 90 seconds, rested, and then repeated the process several times per exercise session. As a result, they burned 225 to 250 calories while cycling, but they burned more fat at the end of the study

---

ABS DIET SUCCESS STORY

MORE ENERGY TO WORK, TO PLAY, AND TO CARE FOR HIS FAMILY

Name: Pete Hemmer

Height: 1.77 m/5'10"

Age: 40

Weight, Week 1: 111 kg/17 st 6 lb

Weight, Week 6: 105 kg/16 st 7 lb

Weight, Week 10: 98.5 kg/15 st 7 lb

Pete Hemmer knew he had to get his body back in order. He had reached 130 kg/20 st and was trying to care for premature triplets. He was unhappy – and out of shape, out of breath, out of energy. 'When I stepped on the scale and saw 130 kg/20 st, I said at that moment, "If I keep going where I'm going, I'll be dead by the time I'm 40."' That's when he knew he needed to change, so he just tried adjusting portion sizes and making smart choices about eating. Over the course of about a year and a half, he whittled himself down to 111 kg/17 st 6 lb – still far off from where he wanted to be. Then he read about the Abs Diet and told his wife, Krista, 'That's the diet plan I need.

'I went out that weekend and bought the book, read it in a weekend from cover to cover, and my wife said I wouldn't shut up talking about it,' he says. Then Krista asked him if it was something she could try, too. On Monday, they made their plan, and on Tuesday, they started.

'As I was pushing the shopping trolley down the aisle, I noticed there weren't any boxes in my trolley. It was fresh vegetables, dairy and

than the workers in group one. In fact, even though they exercised less, their fat loss was nine times greater. Researchers said that the majority of the fat-burning took place after the workout.

So instead of asking you to spend 30 minutes on a stairclimber

---

meat, and there were no frozen pizzas. All the stuff that had become staples of our diet were missing,' he says. 'It was just something that struck me – that even though we had been doing well for a year, there was a lot of room for improvement.'

Hemmer, whose goal was to be in better shape by his 40th birthday than he was at his 30th, instantly saw results – in fat loss and in energy levels. 'I noticed when I was going up the steps to a loading dock, I went up two steps at a time and I didn't even blink, and I realized I had never done that. I just felt lighter.' After the first 2 weeks, Krista even made the comment that they had eaten better the past 2 weeks than they ever had before in their 12 years of marriage.

The rewards kept coming: Krista has lost 6.8 kg/15 lb and a dress size, Pete's down from a nearly 44-size trousers to almost a 34, it's easier to take care of the kids, friends who haven't seen them in months don't even recognize them, and they're even planning a sea kayaking trip. 'That wouldn't have happened before,' Hemmer says. 'For us, sitting on the sofa and watching a pay-per-view movie was the extent of our physical activity.'

When he went to the gym to have his body composition checked after 6 weeks, the woman who ran the machine looked at Hemmer's 6-week improvement and asked him what he was doing. 'I told her briefly about the Abs Diet, and she said that even the gym's weight-loss programme doesn't get such good results,' Hemmer says. 'She also said that it appeared that my body had become efficient at burning fat. I told her politely that it was sort of the whole point.'

And, of course, there's also one other side effect: 'Our sex life has improved dramatically,' Pete says. 'Krista says that if I get in any better shape, she's going to need smelling salts.'

or a stationary bike every day, I want you to add one simple interval workout per week to complement your strength training. Your mode of transport isn't important, so pick whatever activity you prefer. What's important is making sure you change gears. You can vary it in whatever time frames you want (1-minute high-intensity, 1-minute low-intensity, or maybe build up with 30 seconds of high, rest, then 45 seconds, then rest, and so on). Always warm up and cool down for at least 5 minutes at the beginning and end of each interval workout.

Sample Workout Schedule

You'll do circuit training 3 days a week, making sure you have at least 1 day of rest in between days. Additionally, do an interval workout 1 day a week. You also have the option of doing light cardiovascular exercise (cycling, walking, swimming, tennis or golf without the cart) on your off days. On these days, make having fun your main goal – don't think about calorie burns, afterburns, George Burns or any other kind of burns.

Monday: Circuit Training
Tuesday (optional): Walking at brisk pace or light cardiovascular exercise
Wednesday: Circuit Training
Thursday (optional): Walking at brisk pace or light cardiovascular exercise
Friday: Circuit Training
Saturday: Interval Workout
Sunday: Off

The Abs Diet Workout Worksheet

Like naked bodies, all workouts are not made alike. If you're currently not exercising, then anything is better than a nightly chips festival on the love seat. But for the most powerful workouts for burning fat and adding muscle, follow the Abs Diet Workout Worksheet.

Your goal here is to amass a total of 40 points per week. For each activity, you get full credit for doing the activity continuously for 20 minutes. Exercises in the Abs Diet Workout give you the highest number of points, but if you can't keep to that workout schedule, you can sneak in a few extra points here and there to make your workout work. Don't try to go over 40 points a week, though – there's no extra credit for total exhaustion.

10 POINTS (FOR EACH 20 MINUTES SPENT)

Abs Diet Circuit	Interval Training (solo sport: running, swimming, cycling or machine)
Abdominals Circuit	

6 POINTS (FOR EACH 30 MINUTES SPENT)

Abs-specific classes	Mountain biking, intermediate to advanced, hilly course
Basketball (full-court)	
Boot Camp classes	Pilates, advanced
Boxing	Power lifting
Bull running, Pamplona	Snowshoeing, hilly
Calisthenics: press-ups, pull-ups, sit-ups	Spinning classes
	Sports-conditioning classes
Cross-country skiing, hilly	Stairclimbing, stadium stairs
Hiking, hilly	Strength training, non-circuit
Hockey, inline or ice	Volleyball, beach, competitive

4 POINTS (FOR EACH 30 MINUTES SPENT)

Basketball (half-court)	Downhill skiing, intermediate to advanced
BOSU classes	
Dodgeball	Kickboxing classes
Inline skating, steady	Martial arts

4 POINTS (FOR EACH 30 MINUTES SPENT) (CONT.)

Pilates, beginner	Strength-training, ultra-light weights
Racquetball	
Rowing machine, steady pace	Surfing
Rugby	Swimming, steady pace
Soccer	Tennis, competitive
Step classes	Ultimate Frisbee
Strength-training, resistance bands	Volleyball, indoor
	Yoga, advanced or power

3 POINTS (FOR EVERY 30 MINUTES SPENT)

Adventure racing	Kayaking/canoeing
Cross-country skiing, flat	Rock climbing
Cycling, road, steady pace, flat	Snowboarding
Dance-aerobic classes	Stairclimbing machine, steady pace
Downhill skiing, easy	Tennis, recreational
Fishing, big-league tuna	Urban Rebounding classes
Golf, without cart	Volleyball, beach, recreational
Hiking, flat	Walking, brisk
Jogging, steady pace	Yoga, beginner

2 POINTS (FOR EVERY 30 MINUTES SPENT)

Basketball, solo	Ice skating, recreational
Bowling	Softball
Fishing, recreational	Stretching, general
Frisbee golf	Walking, slow
Gardening	Water aerobics classes
Golf, driving range	Wrestling, with kids
Golf, with cart	Yoga, meditative

ABS DIET FAQ

How does the Abs Diet differ from other diets?

Following most popular diet books is like sending your body to prison – they're all about deprivation and restriction. These diets may work in the short term by shackling you to keep you away from certain foods and calories. But once you get a sniff of freedom (in the form of fries and shakes), you're more likely to try to escape. And you know the severe penalties for trying to escape – a life sentenced to a fat gut.

The Abs Diet is about gaining, not restricting. You gain a leaner, firmer body, more control over your life, and even more opportunities to enjoy the foods you love. By eating six times a day, you'll keep your energy levels high and your hunger always at bay, while training your body to burn calories and make itself lean. You'll feed yourself the foods that force your body to lose weight, to burn more calories.

What about really popular ones, like Atkins and South Beach?

The Atkins Diet eliminates practically all carbohydrates for the first part of the plan, leaving you with only foods that contain protein and fat. It's a gimmick that works – in the short term. By restricting the foods you eat to only a handful of them, you'll automatically lose weight because you've dramatically reduced your total calories. But you'll also dramatically reduce your intake of vitamins, minerals and fibre, while upping your intake of artery-clogging saturated fats. The one good thing about Atkins: it eliminates empty carb calories like doughnuts and Doritos. But on the Abs Diet, you dump the lousy carbs and keep the healthy and delicious ones (wholegrain bread, cereal, fruit, vegetables), which will keep you full, fuel your body and dampen your cravings.

The South Beach Diet is based on sound principles of healthy nutrition, and it's a pretty good choice for pure weight loss. But the Abs Diet isn't just about losing weight – it's about turning unsightly flab into lean, sexy muscle. That's why, unlike South Beach, the Abs Diet features muscle-building exercise as part of its foundation. Muscle exponentially speeds up the fat-burning process – 455 g/1 lb of muscle requires your body to burn up to 50 calories a day just to maintain that muscle. This plan combines exercise with the foods that most promote muscle growth.

There are many diets out there today, and as long as people have the opportunity to choose a course for better health, that's what ultimately counts. Frankly, I hate the word *diet* because diet implies that you have to eliminate and restrict, but to call this the Abs Nutritional Superiority Plan seemed a bit much.

How much weight will I lose?

I can't give you a firm number, because people's bodies have more variables than a calculus textbook. I can tell you that some people who have used the Abs Diet have lost 11 kg/25 lb in 6 weeks. That doesn't necessarily mean that you will, but it means that you might or that you could. Much of your success depends on so many factors – including your intensity of exercise and your starting weight. But we've seen a lot of people who've lost between 4.5 and 6.8 kg/10 and 15 lb in the first 6 weeks while also gaining a few kilograms of muscle, which helps them keep burning fat after that initial 6-week surge.

What percentage of body fat do you have to get to so that you can see your abs?

Finding your abs might feel as daunting as digging through sand to find a buried treasure. But if you dig diligently enough – and by that I mean burning off that extra, unwanted flab – you will find the treasure. As far as the specific body-fat percentage, it varies. I've seen both men and women with body-fat percentages in the teens with defined stomach muscles. For most men, you need to get to around 10 per cent. The good news is that if you're exercising regularly, then at least 80 per cent of every 455 g/1 lb you lose will be fat.

Will it work for women?

Absolutely. It doesn't take a Peeping Tom to know that men and women have distinct physiological differences, but in this case, what works for a man will also work for a woman. This eating plan revolves around eating foods that are good for everyone, and the exercise plan is about building lean muscle mass, not rugby player muscle mass. The key is not to count calories but to eat six meals a day to keep you properly fuelled. A woman's portion sizes can be a little smaller than a man's, but by eating well-balanced meals with the ABS DIET POWER 12, anyone can lose fat.

So the ABS DIET POWER 12 foods are the only ones I can eat?

Absolutely not. You build your diet around the ABS DIET POWER 12 – and make sure you have several of them at every meal and snack. You can supplement with other foods, but if your meals are centred on the Powerfoods, you'll ensure yourself a well-balanced diet that keeps you satiated and provides you with the ingredients that help keep your body properly fuelled and turn it into a fat-burning machine.

What about portion control? Can I eat any amount I want?

If you're eating these Powerfoods, they should take care of your hunger so that you don't have the physical urge to eat a lot. By doing things like eating six times a day and making sure you get enough fibre, you'll decrease the chance of shovelling enormous amounts of food into your mouth. That said, it's always smart to be aware of how much you eat – especially when you're starting out. You can cover your plate with the ABS DIET POWER 12, but there's no need to pile the food so high that you need planning permission to construct your plate. Let's just say that a height restriction is in effect.

The Abs Diet includes a weekly cheat meal. Does that mean I really can eat anything?

Yes. One time a week, you can eat anything. You want a chocolate eclair? Eat it. You want a burger? Eat it. You want fried alligator?

ABS DIET SUCCESS STORY

HE INSPIRED HIS WIFE – AND HIS SON

Name: Bill and Kathy Bartz
Bill's age: 56
Height: 1.75 m/5'9"
Weight, Week 1: 85 kg/13 st 5 lb
Weight, Week 6: 77 kg/12 st 2 lb
Weight, Week 12: 75 kg/11 st 12 lb
Body-fat percentage, Week 1: 18.7
Body-fat percentage, Week 12: 10.2
Kathy's height: 1.68 m/5'6"
Weight, Week 1: 57 kg/9 st
Weight, Week 12: 53 kg/8 st 6 lb

Last year, Bill Bartz made a New Year's resolution: he wanted to see his six-pack before the end of the year. He had been lifting weights regularly for 15 years, so he had a lot of bulky muscle mass, but he was missing the definition.

'I saw the author on *Good Morning America* on the Fourth of July, and I thought, hmmmmm,' Bartz says. 'So I decided to go to Borders and get the book. I just started reading it and it all made sense. And what I really liked was how it took other diets and blew them apart.'

Eat it. The cheat meal is designed to reward you for good work throughout the week and help keep cravings in check. And what we found is that once people start seeing results, many don't even want the cheat meal – because the ABS DIET POWER 12 satisfy so many different kinds of cravings. The only caveat is that you must limit yourself to just one cheat meal a week. Do it any more, and you might as well be on the Doughnut Diet.

Can I make food substitutions for the ABS DIET POWER 12?

Many of the 12 categories are broad enough to include many different dietary choices. Low-fat dairy includes milk, yogurt and

---

So Bartz decided to jump on the Abs Diet, and the weight jumped off.

'One day, as I was getting out of the shower with a towel wrapped around me, my wife said, "Whoa, that thing is working."' So Bartz's wife, Kathy, joined in, too. With not much weight to lose, Kathy went from 57 kg/9 st to 53 kg/8 st 6 lb.

Bartz took ab-specific classes 3 days a week at the gym, continued lifting weights, and incorporated interval training into his workouts.

But maybe the best outcome of the programme is what it's done for his overall health. He's taking part in a clinical study in which his blood pressure is measured every 6 months. Since he started, his BP dropped from 130/90 to around 115/70. 'When I went there, they were blown away,' he says. 'Right away, they noticed a difference in weight and they noticed a drastic drop in blood pressure. The nurse even wanted the name of the book so she could get one for her husband.'

Bartz has been spreading the word about the Abs Diet – now, he's in competition with his 25-year-old son in a race for the first one to get a six-pack. His son isn't on the Abs Diet – and he's losing out. Bartz says, 'Last Saturday, I sent him a picture and he said, "Dad, that's not you. You found that picture on the internet."'

'I'm not at a six-pack yet, but I'm darn close,' Bartz says, 'and I know I'll have that six-pack for the end of the year.'

cheese, and lean meat can include turkey, beef, fish and chicken, for example. We do offer some substitution examples for different kinds of foods. Even if you're allergic to one category of food – nuts, for example – you can still figure out what ingredient you're missing by not eating that food and make up for it somewhere else. So having avocado or pumpkin seeds can give you the monounsaturated fats found in nuts – without the danger of an allergic reaction. That said, if you do suffer from food allergies, consult your doctor before trying this or any other diet plan.

Some of the smoothie recipes have cooked instant oats. That sounds gross. How does it taste?

Recipes are a little like CD collections – what works for me might not work for you. But from the smoothies I've had, I can't even taste the oats after they're blended – especially when there are berries or chocolate whey powder in them. So be brave and give it a go: oats add bulk to the smoothie as well as the all-important satiating fibre.

What about this issue of targeting body fat? I thought you couldn't spot-reduce.

Well, you can't spot-reduce per se. That's a myth. But when you lose weight on the Abs Diet – particularly if you're doing some moderate exercise at the same time – you'll lower your body fat and will likely notice much of that loss around your midsection, since that's where most of the fat accumulates. And if you are doing ab workouts and strengthening those muscles, then as the fat peels away, you'll begin to see the washboard.

MEASURING YOUR PROGRESS ON THE ABS DIET

EVERY PERSON HAS HIS or her own way of measuring success on a diet. Some measure it by the way their trousers feel. Some measure it by the compliments they receive. Some measure it by the fact that they no longer have to buy two seats when they fly. But if you want harder numbers to know where you stand, here are some pretty good ways to gauge your progress.

Weight. Kilograms lost help give you some idea, but it's an incomplete number because it doesn't take into account the amount of muscle you're going to develop over the course of a plan. Muscle weighs more than fat, so even a dramatic fat loss may not translate into a dramatic drop in body weight.

Body mass index. The BMI is a formula that takes into consideration your height and your weight, and gives you an indication of whether you're overweight, obese or in good shape. To calculate your BMI, the easiest thing to do is use an online calculator, like the one at MensHealth.com/BMI. A BMI between 25 and 30 indicates that you're overweight. Over 30 signifies obesity. BMI has its flaws as well (it doesn't take into account muscle mass, and it also leaves out another important factor — weight distribution, i.e. where most of the fat on your body resides). But for most people, it's a better indicator of progress than body weight alone.

Waist-to-hip ratio. Researchers have recently started using waist size and its relationship to hip size as a more definitive way to determine your health risk. It's considered more important than BMI because visceral fat — the fat that pushes your waist out in front of you — is a leading indicator for diabetes and heart disease. British researchers recently reported that men with waists of 102 cm/40 in or more, and women with waists of 88 cm/35 in or more, are at substantially higher risk for these diseases — up to four times higher.

That's why I want you to concentrate on lowering your waist-to-hip ratio. To figure out yours, measure your waist at your belly

---

ABS DIET SUCCESS STORY

A FORMER KICKBOXER KICKS IT INTO GEAR

Name: Ray and Kim Welborn

Ray's age: 44

Height: 1.72 m/5'8"

Weight, week 1: 85 kg/13 st 6 lb

Weight, week 6: 78 kg/12 st 1 lb

When he was in his twenties, Ray Welborn weighed in at about 59 kg/9 st 4 lb — it was his fighting weight as a professional kickboxer. But after he stopped, he started putting on weight. One day recently, he and his wife, Kim, were in a bookshop and saw *The Abs Diet*. They immediately took to it — Ray for what he thought it could do for his body, and Kim because it reminded her of the way her parents brought her up to eat healthily.

Ray, who's lost nearly 9 kg/20 lb, and Kim, who's lost 3 kg/7 lb, follow the weekly meal planner in the original *Abs Diet*. 'That's our bible,' Ray says. 'And we stick to it. We even find that we can't eat as much on our cheat meal because of our shrinking stomachs.'

button and your hips at the widest point (around your bottom). Divide your waist by your hips. For example, if your hips measure 102 cm/40 in and your waist at belly-button level measures 96 cm/38 in, your waist-to-hip ratio is 0.94. You want a waist-to-hip ratio of 0.92 or lower.

Body-fat percentage. Though this is the most difficult for the average person to measure because it requires a bit of technology, it's the most useful. That's because it doesn't just take into consideration weight, but also how much of your weight is fat and how much is muscle. Many gyms offer body-fat measurements, or you can try an at-home body-fat calculator. If you want a simple

With the meals, they adjusted recipes just a bit — so that Kim would eat ⅘ of a portion. That's when she started seeing a change. 'I like it because of the healthy food,' Kim says. 'I used to do Weight Watchers, and they all concentrated just on points — it didn't matter whether it had high-fructose corn syrup in it or not. With Weight Watchers, I was always hungry. With this, I'm never hungry.'

Both Ray and Kim have lost the weight from their bellies, and Ray is seeing muscles he hasn't seen in years, including ones right around his rib cage. 'She really feels it when she cuddles up to me,' he says.

More importantly, Ray *feels* healthier. 'I feel lighter. My knees don't hurt as much any more. With the excess weight off, it doesn't hurt to go downstairs like it used to,' he says. 'And I can tell you. I can bend over and tie my shoes and breathe at the same time. Seriously.'

low-tech test (and this isn't as accurate as what the electronic versions will give you), try this: sit in a chair with your knees together and your feet flat on the floor. Using your thumb and index finger, gently pinch the skin on top of your right thigh. Measure the thickness of the pinched skin with a ruler. If it's 2 cm/¾ in or less, you have about 14 per cent body fat — ideal for a guy, quite fit for a woman. If it's 2.5 cm/1 in, you're probably closer to 18 per cent fat, which is a tad high for a man, but desirable for a woman. If you pinch more than 2.5 cm/1 in, you're at increased risk for diabetes and heart disease.

This last measurement can be the most significant because it'll really help give you a sense of how well you're sticking to a plan. As you see your body-fat percentage decrease, you'll see an increase in the amount of visible muscle. Experts say that in order for your abs to show, your body fat needs to be between 7 and 10 per cent. For the average slightly overweight man, that means cutting body fat in about half. If you want to see your progress, take measurements every 2 weeks or so — and certainly not every day.

MEASUREMENT	START	END OF WEEK 2	END OF WEEK 4	END OF WEEK 6
Weight				
BMI				
Waist-to-hip ratio				
Body-fat percentage*				

*Make sure to have the same person administer body-fat readings using the same method to ensure consistency.

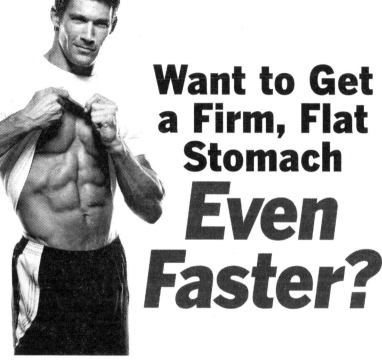

ATTENTION *ABS DIET* READERS!

Want to Get a Firm, Flat Stomach Even Faster?

Log on today and check out amazing Abs Diet tips that will make the body of your dreams a reality.

Guarantee your success with the Abs Diet online programmes. Plus, discover more Abs Diet breakthroughs and the stories of men and women who have made The Abs Diet a success.

Go to:
www.absdiet.com